P9-BUI-664

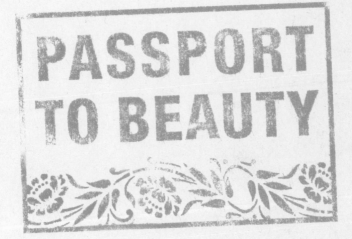

PASSPORT
TO BEAUTY

PASSPORT TO BEAUTY

Secrets and Tips from Around the World for Becoming a Global Goddess

SHALINI VADHERA, CELEBRITY
MAKEUP ARTIST

ST. MARTIN'S GRIFFIN ≈ NEW YORK

www.stmartins.com

Design by Charles Kreloff

Library of Congress Cataloging-in-Publication Data

Vadhera, Shalini.
    Passport to beauty : secrets and tips from around the world for becoming a global goddess / Shalini Vadhera.
        p. cm.
    ISBN 0-312-34962-9
    EAN 978-0-312-34962-2
    1. Beauty, personal—Cross-cultural studies.   2. Women—Health and hygiene—Cross-cultural studies.   3. Skin—Care and hygiene.   4. Herbal cosmetics.   I. Title.
RA778.V18 2006
646.7'042—dc22   2005033036

10   9   8   7   6

This book is dedicated to my mother and father,
for showing me the world with love
and teaching me to appreciate everything it has to offer;
and to Matthew,
for dreaming my dreams with me, every day of our lives.

Contents

Acknowledgments

Through years of research and passion, *Passport to Beauty* became a reality with the help and support of many people, all of whom mean the world to me.

With many, many thanks and deep appreciation to my partner in crime, Cheryl Fenton, who took my words and gave them life, and who made me laugh through the entire process.

To my agent, Andrea Barzvi, thank you for believing in my dreams and passions, and for giving me the opportunity to share my message.

A very special thank-you to Sheila Curry Oakes, my editor, for your constant support, and for sharing my vision in producing this book.

To my family—Matthew, Mom, Dad, Nony, and Neville—thank you for your endless support, countless blessings, and for making me believe that anything is possible.

To my mentor and dear friend Tom Bergeron, thank you for teaching me to never give up, and for opening the doors that allowed me to pursue my dreams.

To Paul Bowers, who so patiently put up with me writing my book—on the job—every time he hired me as a makeup artist. Thank you!

A special thank-you to Marc Tule, www.marctule.com, for your amazing eye for lighting and for shooting such beautiful photos for the cover.

To my champions, teachers, and sweet friends—Marilyn

Grant, Rob Morhaim, Jody Lawrence, Teresa Evans, Paris Heffner, Dr. Joe Platania, Henry Winkler, Harris Jerdon, Babette Perry, Brooke Bryant, Howard Lapides, Mark Turner, and so many more, thank you for your support and for your help in making my dreams a reality.

To my Henna and Rajah, thank you for keeping me company, and for giving me constant unconditional love.

To the men and women I met all over the world, thank you for giving me a glimpse of your culture and for bringing me into your life, and for so enthusiastically sharing your tried and true traditions and beauty secrets. This wouldn't have been half the fun if I hadn't been able to share this experience with you.

With special thanks and great appreciation to the following for contributing their secrets to *Passport to Beauty:*

Marni Abdulhalid (Singapore)

Anda Spa (Phuket, Thailand)

Helle Bagh (Denmark)

Ben (Vietnam)

Sue and Mark Birmingham, Aura Sunspa (New Zealand)

Yelena Blumin, Yelena Spa (San Francisco; Russia)

Centara Spa (Bangkok, Thailand)

Simone Chen, Angsana Spa and Banyan Tree Spa (Thailand; Singapore; Indonesia)

Agnes Cohen (France; Morocco)

Jason Cook, Aurora Spa Retreat (Melbourne, Australia)

Suzette Crawford (South Africa)

Patrizia Deloof (Belgium)

Nita Deshpanda (India)

Meike Devroey (Belgium)

Teresa Evans (China)

Makda Fessehaie (Eritrea)

Alex Forte (Dominican Republic)

Daniella Garcia, Westin Resort and Spa (Puerto Vallarta, Mexico)

Hilda Gardiner (Puerto Rico)

May Hung, dynasTEA Club (San Francisco; China)

Meenu Jasuja (India)

Diane Kern (England)

Esther Kim (Korea)

Koray, Mete Turkmen Hair (Turkey)

Natalie Kosson (Morocco)

Darcy Jensen (Denmark)

Gene Johnson (Egypt)

Elisabeth Longoria (Mexico)

Marlin Marin (Venezuela)

Jacqueline Mgido (Zimbabwe)

Kate Monaghan (Ireland)

Warden Neil (New Zealand)

Mary O'Mally (Australia)

Siham Omar (Ethiopia)

Juliana Ordorica (Zacatecas, Mexico)

Marcella Ordorica (Mexico)

Manjiri Phadris (India)

Rahel (Ethiopia)

Daniela Rizzo (Brazil)

Doina Sandulache (Romania)

Claudia Starkey, Remedix natural skin care (Boston)

Flavia Stingelin (Brazil)

Joette Thompson, Westin Hotel Spa (Grand Cayman)

Tonsai Village Resort (Ko Phi Phi Island, Thailand)

Anocha Uahwatanasakul (Thailand)

Maggie Vasilyadis (Greece)

Rocio Villareal, El Careyes Resort (Careyes, Mexico)

Last but definitely not least, to all my viewers, followers, readers, and visitors to my Web site, thank you for your e-mails, your comments, and your questions, all which have inspired me to take your most requested beauty secrets and turn them into a book—*Passport to Beauty*.

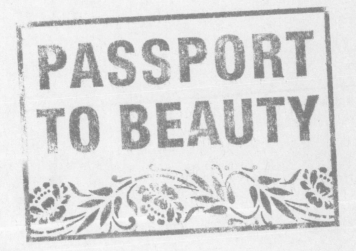

PASSPORT
TO BEAUTY

Introduction
The Journey

As a self-professed beauty junkie, ever since I was a little girl I have been obsessed with watching what women around the world do to look and feel beautiful. From watching them rim their eyes with black kohl liner for a sexy, sultry look to slathering their faces with egg yolk and lemon for an instant facelift, how women stay beautiful has completely mesmerized me!

Having grown up as an Indian-American, I'm no stranger to trips around the globe, with new cultures and histories on the horizon. I have traveled to visit relatives overseas; Africa, Asia, and Europe were just a few stops on our family vacations. One of my fondest memories is flying on the Asian airlines. The Asian flight attendants were some of the most glamorous women I had ever seen. I'll never forget sitting in awe, staring at the beauty of the flight attendants of Singapore and Japan Airlines. They were absolutely perfect, from their flawless makeup down to their perfectly polished toes. I wanted to know everything I could do to look just as beautiful as they did.

I'm not the only one who seemed to take note of their incomparable beauty. On my last trip to Japan, I noticed the flight attendants had come out with their own beauty book, complete with tips on doing your hair and makeup like the crew of Japan Airlines!

With that confession on the table, I think it's safe to say that by the age of eight, my obsession with international beauty had begun.

My love for beauty has led me into a career of helping the already gorgeous become even more so . . . through good skin care and great makeup application. For the past twelve years, I have been lucky enough to work as a makeup artist with countless models and celebrities in Hollywood. It never ceases to amaze me how the right makeup and hair can completely transform someone into an instant glam queen.

THE IMPORTANCE OF A GREAT CANVAS

If there's one thing I have learned over the years, it's that no matter how perfectly you apply makeup, it's hard to disguise bad skin. While hats and scarves can cover up damaged hair, you can't hide for long. If someone is neglecting her skin, hair, and body, the results of flawless makeup are only half of what they could be.

I once worked on a TV show with a young, beautiful actress who had the most stunning facial features. But because she wasn't taking care of herself, you might not have noticed.

Every morning she would arrive with a night of intense partying written all over her face. The bags under her eyes and the condition of her skin were getting worse and worse as the season went on. Finally, the producer asked me if there was anything I could do to help whip this girl back into shape.

The pre-makeup routine is as important (if not more) than actual makeup application when ensuring a fresh-faced look. Every time the actress sat in my chair, she entered a "beauty boot camp." We would start with a cup of warm lemon water for her to drink (this trick helps detoxify the body from the damage inflicted the night before). Then I would apply rose water–soaked cotton pads to her eyes, followed by witch hazel–soaked cotton pads (to reduce the puffiness). We would finish with a great moisturizer. The result? A new, refreshed woman.

TAKING CARE OF YOUR SKIN

How many times have you checked your makeup in the mirror and realized that, even after putting on your face, you actually look ten years older than a glowing example of the true you? It might not be your makeup. It may be that you've neglected your skin for too long, and it's time for some TLC!

Every good makeup and hair routine begins with a good canvas. When was the last time you really took the time to exfoliate the dead skin on your face and hydrate with a great mask? If you neglect to incorporate something as simple as good exfoliation and hydration into your daily routine, you may not be receiving the full benefits of your beauty products. After all, you aren't prepping your skin to accept the full potential of your moisturizer. Your makeup is also most likely grabbing onto the dead skin and simply sitting on top of your face, instead of blending into a flawless finish.

In this day and age, we tend to be obsessed with an easy fix and a quick pick-me-up. We forget that looking great isn't only due to M·A·C's newest shade of eye shadow or CoverGirl's hottest lip color (although those are exciting, too!). Beauty is so much more than skin deep—it's also important to take care of yourself from the inside out.

OUR INTERNATIONAL BEAUTY ADVENTURE

In pursuit of the next best cellulite cream or the latest exfoliant, we completely miss one thing: Mother knows best! Mother Nature, that is. Women around the world have believed in natural remedies to treat and prevent beauty blunders for centuries. In fact, many of these beauty treatments are available right down the street, at your local grocery store!

Every Global Goddess should have a few key ingredients in her beauty pantry.

The Beauty Pantry

Avocado	Olive oil
Coarse sea salt	Sugar
Honey	Lemons/lemon juice
Apple cider vinegar	Beer
Powdered milk	Spring water
Baking soda	Garlic

So if you've ever wondered how Indian women get such lush hair, why Chinese women never seem to age, and how Brazilian women achieve such insane bodies, well, it's not all genetics! They have all benefited from beauty secrets that have been passed down for centuries.

After years of research, thousands of miles logged, and working with some of the best products, I want to share with you the best international beauty secrets I've found. From the Great Wall of China to the lush beaches of the Caribbean, I'll take you on the ultimate beauty adventure around the world. We'll discover and uncover global beauties' top secrets to looking flawless, staying slim, and finding that elusive fountain of youth. I'll also let you in on some of their fabulous makeup tips and share with you some of my own beauty secrets I've used for years on my clients. They are simple enough to become part of your daily beauty routine.

I've also included plenty of recipes. While some ingredients might sound foreign to you, they are usually available at your local international grocery store or ethnic food market.

You may also notice that many of the same ingredients are used in different recipes from all over the world. It's fun to see how countries on opposite sides of the map use the same fruits, veggies, and oils for different beneficial beauty treatments. A few of their tips and ingredients may seem unconventional and odd, but native women swear by them, so have a great time exploring and discovering what works best for you.

My passion for international beauty has inspired me to start my makeup and skin-care line, Global Goddess, which incorporates many of the wonderful ingredients we will be discovering on our journey. Please visit my Web site, www.globalgoddessbeauty.com, for more information on Global Goddess products.

COMMON SENSE RULES

As with any product or treatment, not all treatments are meant for everybody. What may work on one person may not necessarily work on another. I'll never forget the time I used my girlfriend's three-hundred-dollar moisturizer—a rich cream that she swore by. Her skin looked great; mine, on the other hand, broke out completely and turned red. As a beauty junkie and makeup artist, I was in the middle of my worst nightmare! Save yourself this trauma, and be smart about beauty. When trying some of these exotic treatments or adding something new to your beauty routine, listen to your body. If you have sensitive skin or are using something new, do a patch test first to avoid irritation or allergies. You can do this by applying a small amount of the product on the back of your arm or in an inconspicuous area, like the inside of your elbow.

THE BOTTOM LINE

Assess your needs. Don't try everything. Ask yourself if you have a certain beauty challenge and if this treatment promises the right solution. If you're under the care of a dermatologist, then consult him or her before trying something new.

The same is true with makeup. I could never figure out why women would run to the makeup counter at the beginning of every season to buy all the hottest colors and looks. Remember when the "heroin chic" look was really hot? I certainly do. I remember traveling nationally with a makeup artist line and meeting many women in their forties and fifties who were buying all the products to achieve that look. I remember asking a woman why she wanted to look like she had been partying all night and had forgotten to wash off her makeup. She replied by saying she didn't know and just wanted to be hip. Remember, what's hip may not be what's right for you. I always recommend that women choose one set of colors that complements their skin, eyes, and hair. The best way to find this is to go to your local makeup counter and have them show you how to best complement your features. Add a few shades every season to stay current.

Be yourself. Use beauty to enhance your look and not to change who you are. That's the bottom line!

LET'S GO!

I've noticed that no matter the latitude or longitude, women everywhere pride themselves on looking beautiful. Whether we're in Zimbabwe or Beverly Hills, you'd be surprised at how almost all women have the same beauty concerns. They also realize that looking good begins on the inside. Whether it's by starting their day with yoga and meditation or by adding fresh foods to their plate at mealtime, women around the world have always done what they can to look and feel amazing. I have included information on typical diet for each area of our journey, as well as a chapter on travel tips, should you find yourself on a plane to your own exotic destination.

On our quest to becoming a Global Goddess, I'll leave you with this: You'll know her when you see her. A flawless finish, an innate sense of self. She exudes confidence, but knows she can learn from others. She is a curious adventurer, understanding that wherever she goes, something beautiful can be found. She is the true Global Goddess.

Sit back, fasten your seatbelt, and get ready for a trip around the world on your quest to look your absolute best. Enjoy your journey. I know I have!

1

Old-World Charm, Modern-Day Beauty

The first stamp on our passport begins with a journey through old-world charm, Baroque architecture, and cosmopolitan fashion capitals. It's a vacation through Belgium for some hearty beer, down the cobbled streets of France for the finest wines, and to the beaches of the Mediterranean for soaking up some sun and olive oil (not at the same time, of course). It's a European holiday that leaves you looking and feeling like a million euros. From the beaches of Monte Carlo to the Russian Kremlin, we'll discover beauty secrets and tips that make these women the envy of many. Our European adventure is one of artistic beauty, indulgent foods, and fashion trends that demand attention. So get ready, get set, and let's go!

DESTINATIONS

Belgium, England, France, Germany, Greece, Hungary, Iceland, Ireland, Italy, Poland, Romania, Russia, Scotland, Spain, Sweden, and Turkey, to name a few

LOCAL BEAUTIES

European women, known to be some of the most beautiful women in the world, dominate the catwalk and exude confidence with their natural beauty and sense of style. From the smooth, flawless skin of the Nordic beauties to stunning chestnut highlights of the exotic Spaniards, women here use diet as much as natural beauty secrets to gain the upper hand on beauty, as well as gain a sense of well-being.

A TASTE OF THE REGION

Variety is the spice of life, and in Europe, the sky's the limit, but processed food is seen as a huge diet no-no. European women look to their diet to play a huge part in their overall beauty. "You are what you eat" is the universal mantra of many European women. Portion control is another way of life for these stunners. Whether you call it the French Paradox (that magical way French women always seem to stay thin despite all the cheese and chocolate) or just good sense, less is more. Listening to your body is how you best take care of your body. Deprivation leads to failure when it comes to dieting, so instead these gals indulge in all their favorite foods in moderation. Europeans say *oui* or *sí* to chocolate and cheese, but "no" to second helpings. Their trick is knowing when to stop, and not overindulging. Fresh fruits, vegetables, exotic cheeses, fluffy breads, and meats make up most of Europe's menu. While many countries have a signature dish or cuisine, within one country popular dishes may change regionally. Mussels and beer are favorites of the natives of Brussels, Belgium. Exotic delicacies like sheep testicles are saved for special occasions in regions like Iceland. (I may have to pass on that one!) And fish and chips is a must-have in England.

WEATHER REPORT

From the Swiss Alps to the beaches of Monte Carlo, the countries in Europe share a mostly mild climate. With rain and snow seasonally, European climate is cooler than in most other parts of the world. In northeastern Europe, bring your umbrella, because the winters tend to be windy, cold, and gray. Summers are mild, but the sun can hide behind clouds for weeks.

BEAUTY SECRETS OF EUROPE

Europe is one of my favorite places to visit. With countries steeped in history and art, down to the fabulous nightlife and extravagant shopping, it's a must-go destination. I am always struck by how style is visible everywhere. Paris is the beauty capital of the world; Milan corners the fashion market. Natural beauty also makes its mark, as one notices that in certain parts of Europe, many of the women wear little to no makeup at all. Even when keeping the makeup to a minimum, these

European beauties still manage to look great (and healthy!) from head to toe.

A Makeup Remover So Sweet

French beauties treat their skin as delicately as a porcelain vase, especially around the eyes. Their secret to removing eye makeup while hydrating and keeping the eye area smooth? Sweet almond oil. That's right, these gals use a dab of sweet almond oil on a pure-cotton ball to remove makeup around this delicate area.

Shalini's Reminder

Having trouble finding almond oil or any of the other great exotic ingredients in this book? Just take a quick jaunt to your local natural foods store or global market. Most of these items are available in your own neighborhood!

Give Your Feet a Treat

Our feet don't get the constant TLC they deserve, especially in the wintertime. Often neglected, our tootsies are usually left to our pedicurist for all the tough work. It's time to give your feet a treat at home and maintain beautiful-looking toes all year round. Here's a tip from our friends in the Mediterranean, using a traditional staple of many European mealtime dishes—olive oil.

Beautify your feet by dipping them in warm olive oil for a few minutes, and then buff with coarse salt, and rinse. You'll have soft, beautiful feet in no time!

GET DIRTY, GIRL!

As you clean, get dirty! French women soak up toxins with clay, which absorbs oil and impurities without drying or irritating the skin. It draws out toxins from the skin and improves circulation. The best way to find clay is in powdered form at your local natural grocery store. Mix it with a little water (just enough to form a paste), and then smooth it over your face and body. Let dry, rinse off, and feel the difference!

Shalini's Beauty Tip

If you have large pores and a tendency toward dull skin, a clay mask is your answer. It purifies your face, ridding it of dull, lifeless-looking flakes.

Lost Baggage? A Good Thing!

Cucumbers are great for reducing puffiness around your eyes . . . it's a trick that's not so tricky. Just slice a few, and lay them on closed eyelids for a few minutes. One new secret I learned from my friends in Germany was to use chamomile tea bags to get the same effect. Just steep the tea bags in hot water for a few minutes, and let them cool. Place each bag over the eye, and relax for a few minutes. Take them off, and voilà! Your puffiness is gone!

Think Mink for Anti-Aging

And you thought that only the rich and famous wore mink! Wrap your skin in luxury with rejuvenating mink oil. This amazing oil is recommended by many European dermatologists to reduce the look of aging skin. In fact, research by Belgium's Health Department has proven that mink oil is the easiest to absorb and the most compatible oil for human skin. It's perfect for tackling fine lines, wrinkles, and age spots, as well as blemishes, stretch marks, scars, and irritated skin. Use it as a face moisturizer and makeup setter (a few drops of the mink oil spread evenly over your wet face or mixed with foundation), a nourishing treatment for thinning hair (a quick massage with a few drops), and a nourishing bath treatment (1 to 2 teaspoons in the tub).

Shalini's Beauty Tip

If you feel a slight stretching of your skin after applying makeup over the mink oil, not to worry. This is a reaction between your product and the natural mink oil. Eliminate the sensation by applying a moisturizer after the oil.

GRAB THE HONEY, HONEY

Here is some sweet beauty. Polish women apply honey to their faces as an intensive moisturizer. Just a thin layer does the trick. This sweet, golden goo's firming and moisture-retaining properties make it popular with the older ladies as well, while also helping to protect the skin from the damage of UV rays. Smooth it on, then rinse away after a few minutes for softer skin!

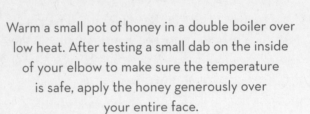

HONEY MASK FOR SENSITIVE SKIN

Warm a small pot of honey in a double boiler over low heat. After testing a small dab on the inside of your elbow to make sure the temperature is safe, apply the honey generously over your entire face.

Leave the mask on for fifteen minutes. It may feel a little sticky, but the moisturizing benefits are worth it!

Rinse thoroughly with warm then cool water.

FEELING BLUE?

Russian women mean business when it comes to keeping their skin healthy looking. Even when their skin is feeling a little blue—black and blue, I mean. They use arnica cream to stimulate white blood cells to fight bacteria around a bruise. The arnica flowers blossom in Russia's Siberian mountains and have tremendous healing power. Although herbal arnica is tough to find, search any natural foods store for topical creams and gels that have arnica as the main ingredient. They do the trick!

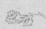 *Shalini's Beauty Tip*

If you're going in for cosmetic surgery, talk to your doctor about taking arnica for a few weeks prior to your procedure. You'll heal faster, and the severity of your bruising will be cut in half.

SCOTTISH SEA KELP

Like a Scottish lass, turn to the sea and restore hair's shine with sea kelp. High in vitamins A, B, C, and E, kelp fortifies follicles and adds shine to hair. The hairdresser's shop is full of several shampoos with sea kelp as a main ingredient. Mix 1 tablespoon of kelp powder and 2 cups of warm water, and massage it into your scalp for two minutes. Then rinse away to fortified follicles!

FRENCH FLOUR FORMULA FOR SHINY, SILKY HAIR

This simple flouring technique is all the rage in France, where women are known for their beauty. This easy formula is the key to lustrous, manageable hair. Evidently, flour smoothes the scales of the hair shaft. *Magnifique!*

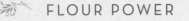

FLOUR POWER

½ cup of white spelt flour
½ cup of barley flour
1 cup of distilled water
1 tablespoon of apple cider vinegar
Shower cap

Sift the flours together in a large bowl. Pour in the water and vinegar, and mix well.

Spoon the mixture onto your dry hair, and smooth the paste all over the hair, avoiding the scalp. (This treatment is for the hair. It's not harmful for the scalp, but the focus is getting the paste on the individual strands of hair.)

Sweep the coated hair up on top of your head, and put on the shower cap. Leave on for twenty to thirty minutes.

Remove the cap and rinse the mixture off hair thoroughly, using cool water. (Hot water will make the flour stick to the hair shafts—a gluey mess!)

Shampoo as usual, rinsing with cool water.

Venetian Gold—The Perfect Hair Color

In Venice, the women once were obsessed with dyeing their hair blond with different concoctions (sometimes using the oddest ingredients, like alum and oriental crocus), choosing the hottest moment of the day to sit outside, and letting the sun bleach away the color. They still knew the importance of keeping skin safe from the sun's harmful rays. These lovelies wore a wide-brimmed hat called a *solana* to protect their faces from the sun while bleaching their hair.

Don't risk your hair's beauty—apply sunscreen on your hair. After all, it needs shielding from the drying summer elements like salt, chlorine, sand, and sun . . . especially if you already have bleached color. Look for sunscreen made specifically for color-treated hair.

Tapped into Beauty

Turn off the tap, and turn instead to thermal water for what your skin needs. French women have started adding thermal water to their skin-care creams and cleansers to help relieve dryness and irritation. This water contains selenium, an anti-inflammatory that gets rid of redness; tap water, on the other hand, can strip away the skin's protective lipids and increase sensitivity.

PERK UP YOUR SUMMER

When summertime hits, Parisian women have nothing to worry about when it comes to perky breasts in their bikini tops! Follow the French and splash on cold water for breast-firming benefits. These flirty women use pulsing, ice-cold shower water to boost circulation, which allows their skin to absorb their favorite breast-firming creams more easily. They also believe that hot baths and steam treatments can cause sagging bust muscles—a definite no-no when it comes to hitting the beach!

A QUICK BRIT FIX FOR WINTER SKIN

Wintertime in England can be harsh on the skin. With whipping winds causing chapping on lips, hands, and any other exposed skin, English lasses ask their local chemist for a glycerin fix for their dry skin. My friend Diane says she and her family swear by glycerin to soften up any chapped areas.

HYDRATE FOR BEAUTY

Scandinavian women know that beautiful skin is just a splash away. These beauties simply drink at least 1½ liters of pure spring water every day, and begin and end their day with 15 to 20 splashes of ice-cold spring mineral water after cleansing, which is said to encourage the skin's own natural functions. In other words, they can skip spending tons of money on expensive skin-care regimens that exfoliate and rejuvenate. The ice-cold water takes care of that for them! Ice-cold water also helps to reduce puffiness while bringing on a rosy glow.

Shalini's Beauty Tip

I love using a spray bottle to mist my clients' faces after applying their makeup. Not only does a light mist help set their makeup, but it also hydrates and refreshes the skin! Try the Global Goddess Refresh Revitalizing Spritzer.

SPICE UP YOUR MOOD

There's nothing like a zesty fragrance to get the heart pumping, the mind going . . . and the mood soaring! Women in Spain know that the trick to elevating their mood starts in the kitchen and ends in the bath. Try enveloping your body at home in this zesty bath, sure to kick up any grumpy day.

SPANISH STRESS-REDUCING BATH

¼ cup of sesame oil
6 cloves
2 cinnamon sticks
1 bay leaf
Dash of dark rum

Combine ingredients. Steep for one hour in a dark glass bottle.

Add three drops to your bath for a lifted mood and conditioned skin.

Lash Out at Lame Lashes!

I used to work with an exquisite model who had the most amazing lashes. She told me about a little secret she picked up in Romania—castor oil. Placed carefully on the eyelashes, it helps to strengthen and stimulate lash growth. It's also good for hair regeneration. Castor oil can rescue your thin, brittle lashes and locks.

Shalini's Beauty Tip

When's the last time you replaced your mascara?
To avoid clumpy, dry lashes and possible eye
infections, make sure to replace your mascara once
every three months. Also, avoid "pumping" your
mascara brush into the tube to get more product
on the wand. By doing this, you push more air into
the tube, causing the product to dry out.

A CARROT A DAY KEEPS THE ACNE AWAY

Hungarian women reach for the carrot to relieve unsightly blemishes and to cleanse oily skin. They dab carrot oil lightly on the offending areas. Women in general have been using carrot oil to treat skin diseases since the sixteenth century. It's rich in beta-carotene and vitamin A, which nourish new cells.

A GOOD WITCH

In England, girls who suffer from oily skin and breakouts turn to witch hazel for skin therapy. Witch hazel, a natural astringent, is used once a day to dry out breakouts and to reduce oil on the face. Make your own oil-control astringent by mixing 1 part witch hazel and 2 parts rose water.

Shalini's Beauty Tip

Witch hazel also reduces puffy eyes. When I'm
working on an actor with puffy eyes, the first thing I
do is reach for the witch hazel. We keep a small
amount in the refrigerator. Soak two cotton pads in
witch hazel, and apply one cotton pad to each
closed lid. Let sit for five minutes, and open to less
puffy eyes.

EUROPEAN FACIAL—A TRUE SKIN TREAT

Nothing says beauty like a facial! Sources tell me that it's the
second most popular spa treatment after massage therapy. After a facial, you leave the spa feeling like you just stepped out
of a glamour magazine. A European facial involves a few basic steps: deep cleansing, skin analysis, steam, exfoliation,
massage, and extraction of blackheads. This routine is followed by an application of products (either a mask or moisturizer) targeted to your skin type, whether it's dry, oily,
mixed, sensitive, or mature. With all that close attention and
special care, your skin will thank you with a healthy glow.

Shalini's Beauty Tip

There are a few things to remember when you have a facial. First, never get a facial the day before a special event. All that massaging and deep cleansing stirs up the impurities in your skin's deeper layers, and you might have a breakout or two. It's also important not to overindulge. Don't have more than one facial a month or every six weeks; your skin needs time to regenerate.

WAKE UP YOUR FEET

Hard day on your feet? Wake up your tired dogs with mint as the British beauties do. The refreshing oils in mint stimulate the circulation and get your toes a-tinglin'. Soak your feet in warm water, then smooth on peppermint oil. Prop up your tootsies on a few pillows, and feel your hard day ebb away. Or mix peppermint oil into unscented body lotion, and give your entire body a minty, refreshing treat!

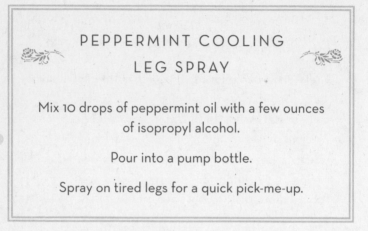

PEPPERMINT COOLING
LEG SPRAY

Mix 10 drops of peppermint oil with a few ounces
of isopropyl alcohol.

Pour into a pump bottle.

Spray on tired legs for a quick pick-me-up.

GET DEEPER COLOR

Brunette beauties in Romania often maintain their naturally
deep, luscious hair color by rinsing with an infusion of wal-
nut tree leaves. The concoction is made by steeping the leaves
in hot water and then straining them out, and it helps to
bring out the hair's dark reflexes. Their blond counterparts
choose a rinse of chamomile tea for golden hair shine.

SWEDISH MASSAGE TO THE RESCUE

A relaxing Swedish massage is all I need to unwind from a
day of the crazies. Traditional Swedish massage was devel-
oped by a doctor in the 1700s and is based on the theory that
by applying pressure and rubbing in the same direction as the
flow of blood returning to the heart, you'll relax the muscles.
This practice uses five main strokes to achieve its relaxing and

healing effects. Through kneading and friction techniques on the more superficial layers of the muscles (so it's not as painful as those deep tissue massages), you will drift away!

Do I Smell Garlic?

If you suffer from goose bumps like I do, you know how hard it is to shave your legs. When savvy girls in Russia cut themselves shaving, they rub cloves of raw garlic on the affected area. Garlic contains antibacterial compounds that help heal those nicks and cuts—fast.

Shalini's Beauty Tip

For a smoother shave, start off your shower with a good exfoliating scrub. Sloughing off dead skin will make your shave smoother, and you'll be less likely to nick yourself.

Lips Like Sugar

Although their moms warm it to use as a supermoist facial treatment, Polish teens use honey to soften their lips. The honey acts as a humectant, drawing moisture from the air to your skin. This balm keeps your lips soft and plump—kissing perfection!

Sugar and Spice Equals Skin So Nice

Sweeten the deal by exfoliating away rough spots the way of the Greeks—with olive oil and sugar. The oil loosens layers of dead skin, while the sugar sloughs them off.

GREEK SUGAR BODY SCRUB

¼ cup of sugar
3–4 tablespoons of olive oil

Mix ingredients to form a thick paste.

Apply liberally in the shower, and massage in a circular motion.

Lighten Your Locks

To brighten their blond hair, German women turn to chamomile. To follow their recipe, add a handful of dried chamomile flowers to a pint of boiling water, and let steep for twenty minutes. Strain, cool, and apply to just-shampooed hair. Let sit for thirty minutes, and then rinse.

LOVE YOUR BLOND HAIR

Speaking of lightening your locks, European beauties know that flowers hold the secret to beautiful blond hair. In Russia, these stunners add a handful of dried daisies to a pint of hot water, and let sit for twenty to thirty minutes. After straining it into a container, they use this floral mix as a final rinse to bring out fabulous blond highlights!

BEER—MORE THAN A DRINK

My girlfriend Patrizia, a fashion stylist from Belgium, has the most incredible sense of style. I had to pick her brain about some Belgian beauty secrets. I asked her about maintaining thick, smooth hair—a definite fashion must-have. She divulged that beer is the secret in Belgium, where there are said to be over four hundred varieties. But rather than drinking it, Belgian women use it as a final rinse for thicker, frizz-free hair.

VINEGAR EQUALS SHINY HAIR

I also spoke with Meike, another talented fashion stylist and Patrizia's mom. She told me that she often uses apple cider vinegar as a final rinse to get super shiny locks. All it takes is ½ cup of apple cider vinegar (available at almost any grocery store). And, of course, you should adjust the amount according to the length of your hair.

The Sour Stuff for Sweet Locks

Seems like these European beauties know a thing or two about shiny hair and apple cider vinegar! In Ireland, women also splash on the tangy vinegar, but it's all they use. That's right, these gals skip the shampoo. Sound yucky? That's exactly what they say for the first week or so, but after that, they don't turn back. They love to flaunt their super shiny locks all over Ireland!

Cocktails, Anyone?

It's all about the cocktail in Spain! The cranberry cocktail, that is! Women of Spain are known for their magnificent hair color. They use cranberry juice to get those fabulous natural highlights! They take ¼ cup of cranberry juice mixed with a ¼ cup of water, and use it as a final rinse.

Shalini's Beauty Tip

If you're blond, make sure you use lemon juice instead of cranberry juice, or else your hair might change color! And pink hair is so not en vogue!

Oil Away Irritated Skin

The Greeks have the secret to soothing irritated skin. These savvy Mediterranean women have been doing it for ages with common olive oil. When they aren't using it for cooking traditional dishes, they are massaging it onto their skin. It's a great antioxidant that helps soften dry, irritated skin. It's also great for treating sunburns. Just make sure you apply it *after* being in the sun, and not while you're sunning. Nobody needs a burn!

Shalini's Beauty Tip

When I'm working on a photo shoot, olive oil is one of my favorite secret weapons to keep in my makeup kit. It works great to tame frizzy hair and fly-aways. Just put a few drops in the palm of your hand, and rub your hands together. Smooth your hand over your hair, and say bye-bye to those pesky fly-aways. Olive oil also works great as a skin luminizer. Just rub it on your legs, shoulders, and arms for glowing, traffic-stopping skin!

INSTANT LEFTOVER LIP GLOSS

After pouring olive oil onto their favorite dish, Italian women rub any oil that they accidentally got on their fingers onto their lips. It gives their pout extra shine and instant conditioning.

Shalini's Beauty Tip

Suffering from dry, chapped lips? There's nothing worse than applying lipstick to rough lips. Talk about a patchy, cakey nightmare. Try this little trick at home: Take an old, soft toothbrush, and apply a small amount of moisturizer to the bristle. Brush your lips gently, and slough off any dead skin. Follow up with a lip balm, like the Global Goddess Drench Hydrating Lip Spa, or a swipe of olive oil before you go to bed. Wake up with soft, smooth lips.

A HEALTHY TAN

Claudia Starkey, the founder of Remedix natural skin care in Boston, told me of a great story of when she was younger, growing up in Romania. At fourteen, she discovered that if she boiled the green shells left over from snacking on walnuts, she could use the liquid concoction as a self-tanning spray. Imagine . . . nature's own sunless tan!

Irish Oatmeal Face Mask

My friend Kate grew up on a farm in Ireland. She told me that for squeaky-clean skin, she and her aunts would make a mask out of oatmeal and milk (oatmeal to soothe and exfoliate the skin, and milk to brighten). Try this mask at home for a shiny, happy face:

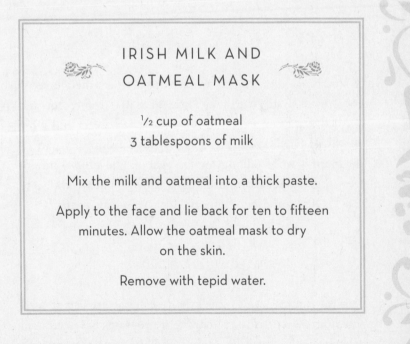

IRISH MILK AND OATMEAL MASK

½ cup of oatmeal
3 tablespoons of milk

Mix the milk and oatmeal into a thick paste.

Apply to the face and lie back for ten to fifteen minutes. Allow the oatmeal mask to dry on the skin.

Remove with tepid water.

Shalini's Beauty Tip

Oatmeal is a soothing treatment for irritated skin, especially if you suffer from rosacea or psoriasis. Just make sure to use oatmeal gently to avoid irritating your skin further and aggravating existing skin conditions. If you're going to try this mask at home, blend or grind the oatmeal for a gentler, softer treatment.

WINE FOR SOFT SKIN

A smashing idea! French women have taken their love of good wine a step further. These gals use freshly cut and mashed grapes on their skin to make it feel softer and more youthful. The linoleic acid and polyphenols in every part of the grape—we're talking the seeds, skin, and pulp—are potent antioxidants with moisturizing benefits and are known to also help fight the aging process. I'll raise a glass to that!

A BEAUTIFUL ROSE

Turkish women love to smell the roses—the essence of rose, rose oil, rose water, rose anything! Rose water has been used as the secret for soothing, toning, and hydrating the skin, and is available at most health and beauty or natural foods stores.

Tone your skin with pure rose water after you cleanse. As an added bonus, replenish your hair's luster by rinsing with rose water. It helps restore shine by sealing the cuticle and softening the look of split ends; plus, you'll smell as pretty as a rose!

 Shalini's Beauty Tip

Does your skin get a little irritated after waxing or threading unwanted hair? Mist your skin with a little rose water after your wax job to help soothe the skin and reduce redness.

FROM PARTY GAL TO POTATO HEAD

In Spain, the nightlife is worth experiencing. Dinners start at 11 P.M., and then it's off to hit some hip, hot nightclubs. When Spaniards sometimes party just a bit too much and end up with dark circles under that eye, they use a potato to lighten the skin. They apply thin slices of potato to their eyes for ten minutes, allowing the juice to seep into the darkness and fade it away. Potatoes contain an enzyme called catecholase, which is used in cosmetics as a skin lightener.

TREATMENT FOR DARK UNDER-EYE CIRCLES

Grated potatoes can also lighten under-eye circles. Run one spud through your food processor, and stuff the raw mash into a piece of cheesecloth. Apply to the area directly beneath your eye—just don't let the potato juice come in contact with the eye itself—and leave for fifteen to twenty minutes. Wipe away the starchy residue.

Shalini's Beauty Tip

Covering a party girl's long night out is nothing new to me. At photo shoots and television shows, it never fails that someone will arrive with evidence of the night before written all over their face. One of the easiest ways to repair a beauty hangover is with concealer. Use a yellow-based concealer a half shade lighter than your foundation. Apply around the eye area and on the lid of the eye with a synthetic concealer brush. Blend lightly with your fingertips. Follow with a few coats of mascara and some pretty pink gloss. No one has to know how hard you partied the night before! Try the Global Goddess Complexion Perfection Duo.

A Real Fountain of Youth

Nothing says relaxation like a soak in a natural hot spring. The ones that run beneath Hungary, known as real fountains of youth, are rich with minerals such as magnesium-hydrogen carbonate, sulfur, and lime, and are thought to heal whatever ails you. The healing pools bubble up nice and hot—perfect for soaking.

To relax away the day in your own home, turn on the Jacuzzi and let the hot water jets massage you. If you don't have the power at home, then treat yourself to a soak in the Jacuzzi at your local spa, or add some Epsom salts to your bathtub.

Shunning the Sun

What's your hurry? Hit the beach a little later to avoid the sun's damaging rays. In Europe, the beaches are deserted between 10 A.M. and 3 P.M. because every savvy sunbather knows that the sun is at its most powerful during those hours.

Rub This, Dry Skin!

In Italy, they mix Mediterranean sea salts with olive oil and rub it all over their bodies. This easy-to-make concoction smoothes away dry flakes and tones and stimulates the skin—while keeping it hydrated.

Shalini's Beauty Tip

Got a nick or cut on your legs? Skip the salt
(talk about rubbing salt into your wounds!)
and opt for sugar.

BEAUTY CAN BE THE PITS!

Munch on tasty Greek olives, but don't toss the pit, say the
savvy Greek beauties. These glamour goddesses keep the olive
stones, grinding them up for use as a body scrub. Ground
olive stones cleanse the body effectively, removing flakes and
dead cells, and providing an immediate glow to the skin.

SOUR SKIN TREAT

In Russia, women adore tanned, bronze skin. But sometimes
too much sun can equal a painful sunburn. My friend Yelena,
from her eponymous spa in San Francisco, told me about a
childhood skin soother she used in Russia. For sunburned
skin, rub cold sour cream onto the burn. Not only does it
soothe your sunburned skin, but the added benefit? It also
helps to brighten the skin as well.

SPEAKING OF LIGHTER, BRIGHTER SKIN . . .

Yelena also gave me a secret for fading those unwanted age and sun spots on your skin. I'm sure that if you have suffered from hyperpigmentation like me, you're always on the hunt for anything that will fade those pesky spots! In Russia, women make a mask of lemon juice and honey (lemon juice to lighten and fade spotting on the skin, and honey to hydrate). Just mix enough together to create a sticky mask, and apply. Leave on for ten to fifteen minutes, and remove with a damp washcloth. You're well on your way to lighter, brighter skin!

Shalini's Beauty Tip

Remember that when lightening your skin, a strict sunscreen regimen is required! You must wear sunscreen every day to avoid having the spotting reappear. I'll never forget the time I had a bout of really bad hyperpigmentation on my jawline. For months I used my lightening creams and sunscreen every day. Then I attended an outdoor wedding and forgot to wear my sunscreen. In an instant, my spotting was back, and I was in front of the bathroom mirror with tears in my eyes. Lesson learned!

Sunny Hair on a Rainy Day

Believe it or not, in Ireland, rainy days can actually mean good hair days. Irish beauties collect rainwater in barrels under their rain gutters. They heat the water and use it to wash and rinse their hair. They swear by this secret for soft, shiny, beautiful hair. In fact, these lasses told, me they have never experienced dry, brittle hair on account of the rain!

Edelweiss Clean and Bright

One of my favorite movies as a little girl was *The Sound of Music*. And who knew that the von Trapp family praised a true skin savior in their famous song "Edelweiss"! Known as the "cloud flower," the tiny white blossoms of edelweiss have brought delicate salvation to faces (and bodies) throughout Eastern Europe with their antioxidant properties. Traditionally, an infusion of the herb was used in the summer to protect from sun (it has natural UV light–absorbing chemicals). To improve the microcirculation, beauties washed their faces with the infusion for a healthy glow. That's music to my ears!

A Moisturizing Desert Flower

Imagine looking to the desert to find moisture! The Spanish prickly pear cactus flower is just that—a miracle of moisture. It contains a high level of water (only cucumber has a higher level), so it's perfect for hydrating tired skin. And there isn't a part of the plant that's discarded; everything is used to replenish moisture. Crushed flowers create an emollient for the skin; a tea made from the leaves is used for hydrating compresses; and the crushed fruit becomes an anti-irritant as well as a moisturizing face mask.

Shalini's Beauty Tip

You can find unique exotic ingredients like the Austrian edelweiss and Spanish prickly pear in the Global Goddess skin-care line. Try the Refresh Revitalizing Spritzer and the Erase Brightening Eye Gel.

DIET TIPS OF THE EUROPEANS

Wherever I go in Europe and whomever I speak to about the diet rules of there, one thing remains constant—these women believe that good food means fresh food.

BE YOUR OWN FIVE-STAR RESTAURANT

Prepare fresh foods at home to control the quality as well as the calories! Processed food is a huge no-no for most beauties in Europe. Their mantra is "you are what you eat." So to keep healthy and slim, be sure fresh foods are on the menu!

Love Your H_2O

A common method of staying slim is drinking tons of water. European women believe in drinking at least 2 liters of water a day to keep their bodies functioning at their best. They also believe in beginning each meal with an ice-cold glass of water to jump-start their metabolism. A glass of water also acts as a great appetite suppressant. Drinking a glass of water before a meal is the perfect way to fill up your tummy and suppress the need for a second helping.

Go Fish!

The typical Mediterranean diet, which consists of mostly seafood and greens, is known for keeping the weight off as well as keeping the body healthy. Choose fish such as mackerel, trout, herring, sardines, albacore tuna, and salmon that are high in omega-3 fatty acids, which are known to benefit the heart and help maintain a healthier you.

Less Is More

Feel like dessert? Then have some! But only a bite. European women believe in eating what you want, but portion control is key. Eat what you love, but don't overeat. Listen to your body, and stop as soon as you're satisfied. Slowing down and taking time to enjoy your meal will help you listen to your body.

Three Meals a Day Is All You Need

In Belgium, women stick to three meals a day and say no to snacking. It's their secret to keeping the scale from tipping in the wrong direction.

SHALINI'S EUROPEAN MAKEUP TIPS

One feature I love about European women (and French women in particular) is how well they wear their makeup. They aren't afraid to use a colorful palette to make a statement. Pull yourself out of your brown and neutral safety zones. Add some color to your beauty routine with these simple steps.

Pick a Feature and Make It Pop

Look at your face. What's your best feature? If it's your eyes, concentrate color on your eyes; if it's your lips, concentrate on your lips. Play it up! Avoid trying to emphasize all your features at the same time. Overdoing it may label you as a makeup misfit!

Toss the Browns—You Want the Eyes to Have It!

In place of your trusty brown eye shadow, try a chartreuse, a light lilac, or a sky blue. Opt for colors that have a slight shimmer or iridescence to them. Bright colors in matte finishes can look flat and may actually age you, so find shadows that have a satiny finish and reflect light.

OK, If You Must Wear Brown

If you aren't ready to toss aside your neutral shades, no problem. You can still incorporate color into your daily beauty routine. Choose a bright color of eye shadow, and apply it from the lid to the crease. Then blend in your brown or neutral shadow through the crease. Keep the rest of your look simple and clean. If you're color shy, opt for a sheer version of your favorite color. That way you can enjoy just a hint of hue.

Start Pouting

Join your French girlfriends and play up your lips with a classic red. Red lips are bold and beautiful. If you're a makeup novice, red can make you feel like you're wearing a lot of makeup. Beware: This color can look easily overdone or cheap if worn incorrectly. Follow these basic rules for pulling off classic red lips:

The Rules of Red

The key to wearing red lipstick successfully is making your lips the feature you want to stand out. Don't wear a lot of other makeup. Keeping the rest of your face natural is the way to go.

In fact, you'll need *less* makeup than you ever have before to feel put together. Skip the heavy eye shadow, blush, brow pencil, and so on. Your face should look clean with light makeup, such as a wash of champagne eye shadow. Add a few coats of mascara. When it comes to choosing an eyeliner, stick with basics, and opt for black, brown, or charcoal colors—only on your top lid.

Red lips pair nicely with a soft bronzer instead of blush. Too much of anything will make you look like a tart!

Groomed eyebrows are an absolute must to pull off red lips. Red lips say "look at me, I'm confident and well put together," and what that means is great-looking brows! (Look to Asia for great tips on getting perfectly groomed brows.)

The Safe Red

Gloss is a subtle way to wear red lips—it's a softer, sheerer look. If you're trying to keep it natural looking, using a liner will take that whole feeling away. If you want longer wear, fill in your entire lip with a nude liner, and then follow with a red gloss. That way, there's less room to make very noticeable lining mistakes!

GOOF PROOF YOUR RED

Light to medium skin looks best in cooler reds, and medium to dark skin looks better in warmer reds. Reverse this rule if you want to add extra drama. Also, red lipsticks tend to bleed more than any other lip color. My favorite way of stopping the feathering is by using a little foundation on a synthetic concealer brush and tracing the lip line. It works as a frame to keep your lipstick in place.

THE RED ALTERNATIVES

Bricks, crimsons, and wines are more neutral versions of the classic red lip color and are more user-friendly. You can tell whether a color is a wine or brick by looking at the undertones. If the red has plum undertones, it's more of a wine; if it has brown undertones, it's more of a brick.

LESS IS MORE WHEN IT COMES TO MAKEUP

Another classic look I noticed throughout Europe was flawless-looking skin. I say "skin" because heavy makeup wasn't apparent in achieving this look. Clean, flawless-looking skin is the secret to staying youthful. It's makeup applied in such a way that it doesn't look like makeup.

One common makeup blunder I see often is the overuse of foundation. We all have areas that might need a little extra help, but that doesn't mean we need to buy the heaviest foundation on the market. I see this mistake being made time and time again, by even the most experienced beauty junkies.

Instead, opt for foundation with a sheerer texture. Apply your foundation first, and then follow with a good concealer to camouflage those areas that need a little extra help. Remember, less makeup is always more flattering to the face and skin.

2

A Journey to the East

The second stamp on our passport of beauty is for taking a trip through time, where women keep the wrinkles at bay. It's a journey through Asia, with adventures in Japan, China, India, Tibet, Thailand, and many other countries in the East. We will discover that inner peace is the key to outer beauty. We will learn the ancient secrets women have used to strengthen hair and to keep their skin flawless and ageless. These beauties will also show you how to turn back the hands of time through daily yoga and meditation.

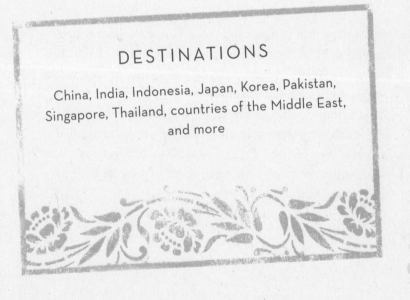

DESTINATIONS

China, India, Indonesia, Japan, Korea, Pakistan, Singapore, Thailand, countries of the Middle East, and more

LOCAL BEAUTIES

In Japan and China, porcelain skin makes these women the envy of all. Throughout Asia, women lighten, brighten, and whiten to achieve the ageless, smooth faces of the Japanese geisha and the wrinkle-free beauties of China. The luxurious tresses of the Indian woman are coveted by those who look to the East for beauty tips. When you also consider the benefits of serenity through meditation, Asia is a fascinating place for both external and internal beauty.

WEATHER REPORT

Asia is the world's largest and most diverse continent, covering about 30 percent of the land area on Earth. It has the greatest range of land elevation of any continent, boasts the longest coastline, and is subject to the world's wildest climatic extremes. This means that from the beaches of Thailand to the dry deserts in the north of India—and all the "tropical deserts" in between—women throughout Asia must battle a range of climates in order to preserve their natural beauty.

BEAUTY SECRETS OF THE WOMEN OF ASIA

POLISH FOR RADIANT SKIN

On a recent trip through Thailand, I absolutely fell in love with the beauty of the country. Lush tropical beaches in the south, old-world history throughout the north, and in the center of it all, Bangkok, a mecca of beauty and fashion. Every international makeup line you could want is available in this capital city's magnificent shopping centers. But even with the availability of modern-day luxuries Thai beauties still rely on age-old treatments for looking absolutely flawless.

My trip started in Phuket, at an ultralush, tropical resort. Sitting on Patong Beach with hundreds of coconut trees and lotus flowers, I was instantly enchanted, and I knew I was going to find some fabulous beauty secrets in this paradise!

My first stop was an exotic spa tucked away a block from Patong Beach. The women who worked there had the most beautiful complexions and soft skin. I needed to know what I could do for my jetlagged, itchy, dry skin. My arms and legs were in dire need of some serious exfoliating, and I knew I had to whip my skin into shape before hitting the beach in my new, little bikini! I asked for a traditional Thai body scrub, not knowing what kind of fabulous treat awaited me! A coconut and jasmine full-body rice polish followed by a Thai massage was just what the doctor ordered!

TROPICAL ESCAPE BODY POLISHER

Rice and coconuts are staples of the Thai diet, but are also used as secret ingredients in many Thai beauty routines. Rice works as an excellent exfoliant because of its gentle but gritty nature, and coconut nourishes the skin with its rich hydrating properties. Try this recipe at home for an instant tropical escape and full-body glow!

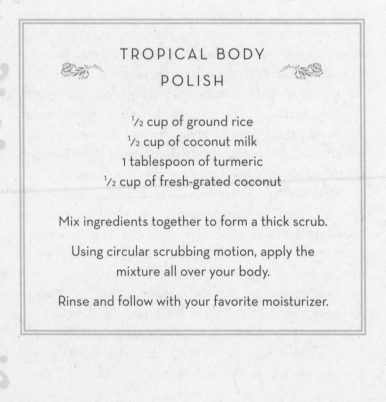

TROPICAL BODY POLISH

½ cup of ground rice
½ cup of coconut milk
1 tablespoon of turmeric
½ cup of fresh-grated coconut

Mix ingredients together to form a thick scrub.

Using circular scrubbing motion, apply the mixture all over your body.

Rinse and follow with your favorite moisturizer.

Shalini's Beauty Tip

Any time you exfoliate your skin, make sure you follow with a good moisturizer to replenish the skin with hydration. When you exfoliate, you must hydrate to avoid overdrying. If you have some time, follow this body polish with a massage using your favorite essential oil. Because coconut is the main ingredient in this scrub, I love to follow it with pure coconut oil rubdown. If you don't have time to make this polish at home, try the Global Goddess Brighten Turmeric Cleansing Body Polish. Use this to exfoliate, and follow with the Shine Coconut Amla Revitalizing Hair Treatment, which can be used all over your body for great moisturizing benefits!

SMOOTH SKIN WITH ALMONDS

It's pure almond oil to the rescue for the women of India. Almond oil softens and gets rid of dry skin in a flash! Use it on your body as a special massage oil before or after your shower or bath, and use a few drops on your face after cleansing at the end of the day.

The best almond oil is made at home, since commercial almond oils have preservatives. Follow my friend Hilda's recipe for creating your own almond oil:

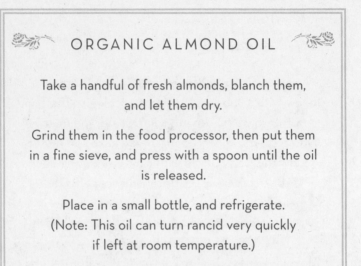

ORGANIC ALMOND OIL

Take a handful of fresh almonds, blanch them,
and let them dry.

Grind them in the food processor, then put them
in a fine sieve, and press with a spoon until the oil
is released.

Place in a small bottle, and refrigerate.
(Note: This oil can turn rancid very quickly
if left at room temperature.)

A Body Brightener

In India we use tamarind as a sauce or chutney on our food. It
has a great sour taste that perfectly complements many dishes
that you can buy right on the streets of New Delhi. In Thailand, they know the benefits that the tamarind fruit lends to
the skin—it's quick way to lighten and brighten, while purifying, exfoliating, and deep cleansing—perfect for Thai women
who live in a culture where light skin is considered beautiful.
Its high acidic base, considered even more acidic than lemons
and oranges, is the centuries-old secret. Because of the numerous skin-care benefits, it's not uncommon to find tamarind
baths and scrubs at spas all over Thailand.

Quenching Flower Power

One of the things I loved about Thailand was the use of fresh flowers everywhere! Whether they are draped in garlands or wearing freshly cut blossoms placed delicately in their hair, women make a beauty statement with flowers! Champak, orchids, and jasmine were a few of my favorites. The scent of fresh jasmine flowers reminds me of walking through the palaces in Bangkok. It's not uncommon for these Thai beauties to soak fresh jasmine flowers in cold water for a soothing summer drink. Delicious, to say the least!

Shalini's Beauty Tip

For a special occasion, wear your favorite flower in your hair. Not only will you smell beautiful, but you'll look fabulous!

Sleep Deeply

In the Middle East, Iranian women love to slumber away to the sweet-smelling bloom of their native jasmine flower. The blossom's fragrance is said to reduce anxiety and create a sense of relaxation. For an amazing night's sleep, place a bowl of heady jasmine potpourri next to your bed and guarantee yourself some heavy z's. Awake with freshness and energy!

Sayonara, *Age Spots*

Follow the lead of the Japanese geisha, women who know flawless complexion. Two drops of camellia oil mixed with a tablespoon of sake is all it takes for clearer, smoother skin. The combination of the two helps to fade freckling, sun spots, and age spots, creating a more even skin tone. In addition, there are incredible moisturizing benefits! You can find pure camellia oil on the Internet through many Asian Web stores.

Shalini's Beauty Tip

If you suffer from hyperpigmentation (a dark discoloration of the skin due to hormonal imbalances, pregnancy, or an adverse reaction to medication), make sure to wear a sunscreen of SPF 30 or higher daily when trying to fade any spots or freckling.

Balinese Papaya Pumpkin Facial

If you have ever visited spas or resorts in exotic locales in Asia, you've probably seen a facialist select and mash fresh fruit for a fresh, on-the-spot enzyme mask. Easy to recreate at home, this mask from Bali will leave your face fresh and glowing.

BALINESE PAPAYA MASK

²/₃ cup of fresh papaya, mashed
15 oz. can of pure pumpkin
1 egg, beaten until frothy

Cut the papaya in half, and discard the seeds.

Scoop out the papaya fruit and mash, and then mix in the egg.

Add the pumpkin and whip together. (Put ingredients in a blender or food processor for an extra smooth mask.)

Apply the mask to a clean face, taking care to avoid the immediate eye area. If you have sensitive skin, test the mixture on your hand before spreading it on your face. You'll feel some tingling as the enzymes in the pumpkin go to work immediately, gently exfoliating your top layer of skin. Leave on for ten minutes, rinse, and follow with a moisturizer.

BE A PRINCESS FOR A DAY

The *lular* ceremony is a traditional Indonesian bridal ceremony that every woman (bride or not) should experience. It begins with the *lular* scrub, combining all the benefits of turmeric, rice, jasmine flowers, ginger, and other spices to help energize the body. It's followed by a yogurt mask to remove the scrub and to prep the skin for the next enchanting step—an exotic flower bath.

For your own exotic flower bath, buy a bagful of flowers or rose petals, and add them to your warm bath water. Flowers are said to soothe the soul and uplift the spirit. Don't just save it for a special occasion—pamper yourself once a month with a different flower.

SAKE: A SKIN SAVIOR

Sake is an all-around miracle worker. This clear rice wine is claimed to be an excellent exfoliant for the face, a great detoxifier for the body, and a tonic that will smooth rough hands and feet. Never mind that it regenerates the skin! Sake is also known to help fade age spots, soothe irritated skin, and ease muscle aches. And I just thought it was a great cocktail with sushi! Add 1 cup of sake to a hot bath for a whole-body detoxification. Bathe for at least ten minutes, and follow with a cool shower. Your skin will feel soft and your muscles relaxed.

FOR A GLOW, THINK MANGO

Thai women use this enzyme-rich fruit to whisk away dry skin and bleach freckles—thanks to the active enzyme papain (it exfoliates) and the antioxidant vitamins A and C (they speed skin repair gently). Vitamin C is a citric acid, so you're getting the same benefits as you would from a glycolic acid, which aids in exfoliating your skin without having to manually scrub it. It will renew your skin cells faster than if you were to use a manual scrub exfoliant.

FLAWLESS-LOOKING SKIN AND STRETCH MARKS BEGONE!

A geisha's flawless complexion can now be yours. The secret of these Japanese lovelies and their smooth skin is camellia oil. White camellia nut oil, used for centuries in Asia, contributes its moisturizing, conditioning, nourishing, and softening benefits to the skin without leaving any oily traces. (It's one of the quickest-absorbing oil out there!) Its high oleic acid content aids in antioxidation, so use it on your face and body for an unparalleled glow. Its special formulation also helps eliminate stretch marks caused by pregnancy, revitalize hair growth, treat burns, and strengthen nails. I know a few celebrities who swear by this oil for combating stretch marks while pregnant. Try the Global Goddess Seduce Face and Body Silk made with pure white camellia nut oil.

Shalini's Beauty Tip

Before bed, massage two drops of camellia oil onto your face in an upward circular motion.

You Glow, Girl!

No one should have a more visible glow than a blushing bride. Indian women make their skin radiant on their special day with a traditional mixture of chickpea flour (an oil absorbant), turmeric (a great anti-inflammatory and antiseptic), and almond oil (talk about moisture!). Their faces and bodies are instantly exfoliated, and skin is softened and brightened.

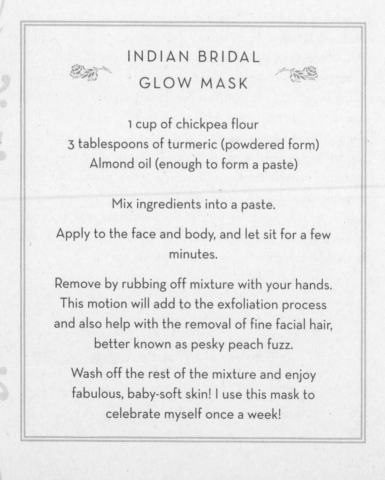

INDIAN BRIDAL
GLOW MASK

1 cup of chickpea flour
3 tablespoons of turmeric (powdered form)
Almond oil (enough to form a paste)

Mix ingredients into a paste.

Apply to the face and body, and let sit for a few minutes.

Remove by rubbing off mixture with your hands. This motion will add to the exfoliation process and also help with the removal of fine facial hair, better known as pesky peach fuzz.

Wash off the rest of the mixture and enjoy fabulous, baby-soft skin! I use this mask to celebrate myself once a week!

SAY BYE-BYE TO STRETCH MARKS

If you're pregnant and want to avoid unsightly stretch marks, follow the advice of Indian lovelies. Mix 1 cup of plain yogurt with 1 tablespoon of turmeric, and apply the paste onto your stomach and waist. Leave it on for ten to fifteen minutes, and then jump in the shower for a quick rinse. These gorgeous women swear by this potion to keep their skin smooth and supple, and to combat stretch marks when baby is on its way.

YOUR INCREDIBLE SHRINKING PORES

At the Banyan Tree Spa in Singapore, these beauties know that a flawless complexion is the trick to great-looking makeup. They create wonderful masks that help to remove blemishes, lighten the complexion, tighten pores, and soften skin. Sounds like a miracle mask to me! Of course, after seeing how beautiful the women were in Singapore, I was the first person in line to try it.

BANYAN TREE
FACE MASK

1 tablespoon of oatmeal
$\frac{1}{3}$ teaspoon of turmeric powder
1 teaspoon of honey
$\frac{1}{2}$ teaspoon of milk powder
1 tablespoon of hot water

Add hot water to the oatmeal and mix well.
Follow with the remaining ingredients.

Gently massage the paste onto the face, and
leave it on for ten minutes before rinsing off.

Shalini's Beauty Tip

If you're like me and breakouts leave nasty dark
spots on your face, the Banyan Tree Face Mask can
be a face saver. Remember that when doing any
type of lightening to the skin, you must wear a
sunscreen that's at least an SPF 15 on your face
every day; otherwise, your dark spots will reappear
after some time in the sun.

Brighten and Tighten Your Face

Flight attendants for Singapore Airlines have to be some of the most beautiful women I have ever seen. On my last trip to Singapore, I was getting ready to leave my hotel in New Delhi when an entire flight crew walked into the lobby. After a long international flight, they still looked fabulous! I had to get their beauty secrets, so I walked over and pleaded with them to tell me. In exchange, they wanted the scoop on the shopping secrets of New Delhi. We had a deal! Flight attendant Marni Abdulhalid had the most radiant skin. She told me a secret that had been passed down from her grandmother—an easy way to achieve radiant skin in no time.

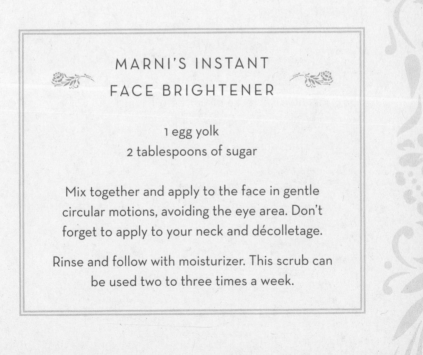

MARNI'S INSTANT FACE BRIGHTENER

1 egg yolk
2 tablespoons of sugar

Mix together and apply to the face in gentle circular motions, avoiding the eye area. Don't forget to apply to your neck and décolletage.

Rinse and follow with moisturizer. This scrub can be used two to three times a week.

BEAUTY THAT COMES NATURALLY

Henna has safely and beautifully colored and conditioned the hair of Indian, Pakistani, and Middle Eastern women for thousands of years. It's another beauty tip that has been in my family for generations.

The leaves of the henna plant are dried and then used for hair color. The tannin from the leaves binds to the keratin (hair) molecules and makes the fibers stronger, enriching the color. After you apply henna to your hair, you'll notice that your hair is softer and stronger, with fewer tangles and sealed cuticles, which reduces the appearance of split ends.

Shalini's Beauty Tip

Add black tea or coffee to the henna mixture. The acidity of the tea or coffee will make the color stronger and richer.

Shalini's Beauty Tip

Never put henna on hair that has been chemically treated within the last year. (Chemical treatments include bleaching, coloring, perming, and straightening.) Henna and chemically treated hair equals disaster! If you are a blonde or a light brunette, look for henna that doesn't deposit color. You can find a clear gloss henna at most beauty supply stores.

DO CHINESE WOMEN EVER AGE?

We all know the benefits of green tea, but in China white tea is the quintessential anti-aging secret! Also known as the emperor's tea, white tea comes from the silver tip of the green tea plant, and is one of the strongest antioxidants in the world. Consider it a suit of environmental armor—free radicals (pollutants in the environment that can damage skin) bounce right off! It's great for reducing puffiness and firming the area around the eye. Recently, a few skin-care lines have realized the benefits of white tea and have begun to incorporate it in their products.

CHINESE WHITE TEA ANTI-AGING MASK

2 tablespoons of brewed white tea
½ cup of green tea powder (or enough to form a thick paste)
4–5 drops of lemon juice

Mix the white tea with the green tea powder.

Add the lemon juice, and mix to form a paste.

Apply to the face and neck, and leave on for five to ten minutes.

Wash off with lukewarm water.

Try Bitter for Better Hair

In Vietnam, women know the secret to strong, healthy hair. They simmer fresh lemongrass in boiling water for ten to fifteen minutes. After letting it cool, they use this bitter wash as a final rinse for strong, healthy, shiny hair.

INSTANT HAIR LUSTER

Filipina women add luster to hair with aloe. These light green, speckled stalks line a well-known path to nourishment. The gel-like molecules help hair reflect light, while the numerous vitamins and minerals including vitamins C, E, and zinc help fortify hair shafts. Apply fresh aloe gel to the hair as a mask before shampooing once a week.

THE SEXY, MYSTERIOUS EYES OF INDIA

Take advice from Indian beauties for a sultry gaze sure to mystify. Indian women dip a wet stick into black powder known as *kajal* or kohl (or use a kohl stick) and line the inner rims of their eyes. They also believe that applying *kajal* behind the ear will ward off the evil eye. Keep in mind that the "kohl" pencils sold in drug stores are not necessarily the real thing, so look for genuine kohl at Arab or Indian specialty stores.

Shalini's Beauty Tip

A deep, rich black eyeliner color is the easiest way to glam up your eyes and create a dramatic flair. A definite must-have for every woman.

Shalini's Beauty Tip

Save your black liner for evening glamour. Black looks better for a more dramatic style, as it can look too harsh for everyday wear and adds years to your look.

THE (COLORED) EYES HAVE IT

To add to their mystique, the hip and trendy women in the major cities of India and in Bollywood change their eye color with colored contacts. I love the possibilities!

It's a great way to really play up your eyes, experiment with different eye shadow colors, and change your hair color. I love to change my brown eyes to gray or green whenever I have a fun event, or just to mix up my beauty routine. I also noticed I can get away with a darker hair color when I wear gray and green lenses. You'll be amazed at how many more colors you can incorporate into your makeup palette. Colored contact lenses are a beauty must-have for any and every season! If you need prescription lenses, visit your eye doctor to experiment with the different colored contacts. Non-prescription lenses are available in most eyeglass stores or online.

Make Light of Your Skin

Light skin is valued just about everywhere in Asia. But in Korea, they don't spend a fortune on skin whiteners to achieve the light look. After soaking white rice to ready it for cooking, Korean women use the starchy, milky water to wash their faces. The result is lighter-looking skin and a soft, dewy complexion.

Scrub-a-Dub Dead Skin

In southern Thailand it's salt and sand to the rescue. On my way to shop at the floating market (about three hours outside of Bangkok), I was fascinated by hundreds of mysterious heaping white mounds on the roadside. The scenery was blurred by my driver's hurried pace (not uncommon in Thailand!), so I couldn't really tell what the Thais were harvesting. Since these farms were in water and there were heaps and heaps of white being pulled out, I automatically assumed the mounds were rice. I finally made the driver pull over so I could investigate. They turned out to be none other than heaps of fresh salt. Unbeknownst to me, I was venturing through Thailand's famous salt farms.

I asked a few nearby women if they used all the salt for cooking or something else. One lady laughed and told me that their secret for ultrasmooth and exceptionally soft skin was a body scrub made from a mixture of coarse, natural salt and sand from the southern beaches. They know that removing dead skin is the secret to beautifully glowing skin!

For your own sand and salt body scrub to reenergize and

get enviable, smooth baby-soft skin, use the following ingredients, and scrub-a-dub dead skin buildup.

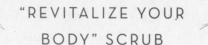

"REVITALIZE YOUR BODY" SCRUB

½ cup of sea salt
½ cup of beach sand
A few drops of your favorite essential oil

Mix ingredients into a thick, paste-like scrub.

Step in the shower and apply in circular motions all over your body. Concentrate on rough areas like the bottoms of your feet, heels, elbows, and knees.

Rinse and follow with a rich body lotion.

SHINIER-THAN-SHINY LOCKS

In India's very cosmopolitan city of Bangalore, it's common knowledge that the secret to ultrashiny locks lies within the delicate white petals of the hibiscus. Dry these beautiful flowers, and boil them with coconut oil. Apply the oil once a week, and leave on overnight. Wash in the morning, and walk out of your bathroom with jaw-dropping, shiny hair. You may want to lay a towel over your pillow to keep your linens clean.

KEEP ACNE AT BAY

Another one of Marni's grandmother's secrets helps her control acne and whiteheads. Try this mask at home to reduce whiteheads and tame a too shiny face.

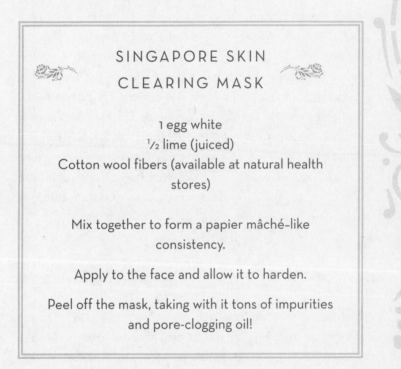

SINGAPORE SKIN CLEARING MASK

1 egg white
½ lime (juiced)
Cotton wool fibers (available at natural health stores)

Mix together to form a papier mâché–like consistency.

Apply to the face and allow it to harden.

Peel off the mask, taking with it tons of impurities and pore-clogging oil!

LUSH LOCKS OF INDIAN BEAUTIES

With such shiny tresses, Indian women should rub it in . . . coconut oil, that is. It's the trick to getting full, thick, shiny hair. It's also great for strengthening thinning hair. For to-die-for shiny hair, Indian women give themselves a hot coconut oil scalp massage once a week to promote growth and wash away tress stress. Coconut oil is one of the richest oils in the world, and it's great for making hair shiny, strengthening follicles, sealing the cuticles, helping with split ends, and stimulating hair growth.

Growing up, my cousins and I lined up to get a good old scalp massage from my grandmother. Enlist the help of a friend or loved one for your own bit of heaven. It makes the treatment that much better! Put some coconut oil in a bowl (it's available at your local Indian store, or try the Global Goddess Shine Coconut Amla Revitalizing Hair Treatment), and give yourself a scalp massage once a week. Sleep with it on, and wash in the morning! Again, I always like to lay a towel over my pillow to keep my pillowcase from getting oily.

Let's not discount the rest of your body. Coconut oil can also bring an amazingly dewy moisture to your skin, wherever you rub it in.

THREAD LIGHTLY FOR AMAZING EYEBROWS

Shaving and waxing generally works for getting rid of pesky, unwanted hair, but for the women in Asia and the Middle East, threading is their choice for becoming fuzz-free. Originating in Arabia and South Asia, threading involves creating a mini-lasso and twisting and pulling along the area of unwanted hair as it lifts the hair follicle directly from the root. The ouchless factor aside, threading also lasts longer than waxing. It doesn't pull on the skin or cause trauma to the skin or follicles. Known for its precision, this method gives the most amazing-looking eyebrows. I highly recommend it!

Shalini's Beauty Tip

If you have sensitive skin like me and tend to break
out from waxing, threading is a great alternative to
hair removal. Find an expert threader who moves
quickly for painless hair removal.

GIVE YOUR HANDS A HAND

For centuries, Japanese rice makers noticed that the hands of
people who washed rice were always super smooth. Japanese
women take this stumbled-upon trick to heart, splashing rice
water on their skin for incredible softness.

WAKE UP YOUR SKIN

Coffee is a revitalizing way to wake you (and your skin) up in
the morning! Indonesian women brighten their skin with a
scrub of coffee grounds. It exfoliates, and the aroma is proven
to elevate moods. Coffee is also used in the treatment of cellulite, and the natural acids help tone and exfoliate tired skin
and improve cell metabolism. The result? Skin so soft and
silky!

Solving the Dandruff Doldrums

In India most beauty secrets start in the kitchen. *Methi,* a spinach-like vegetable also known as fenugreek, is one of the healthiest staples of the Indian diet, known to aid digestion and help with allergies. Within its dark green leaves also lies southern India's secret to keeping dandruff at bay. Here are two great tips from my Indian friend Manjiri using the plant's seeds, which are available at your local Indian grocery store:

1. Boil fenugreek seeds with coconut oil. Apply and massage mixture onto the scalp. Wrap your head in a shower cap, and leave on overnight. Wash your hair in the morning.

2. To treat a dry and itchy scalp, soak the fenugreek seeds for a few hours, and grind them into a paste. Apply to the scalp one hour prior to shampooing. The paste will soothe an itchy scalp and help control dandruff.

Fountain of Youth

White clay is the hush-hush way Burmese women maintain their youthful-looking skin. Mixed with special herbs and green tea, it helps restore softness and wakes up tired-looking skin. If you can't find white clay, try a purifying clay mask once a week. For optimum results, apply at the beginning of your shower, and allow the steam to open up your pores. Rinse off toward the end of your shower, and you'll have an instant facial! Your skin will look softer, and your makeup will glide right on.

TIGHTEN AND TONE

Image-conscious Korean women love to use products from the pantry for more toned, firm skin. My Korean friend Esther shared with me her family's secret for a great pore tightening facial mask:

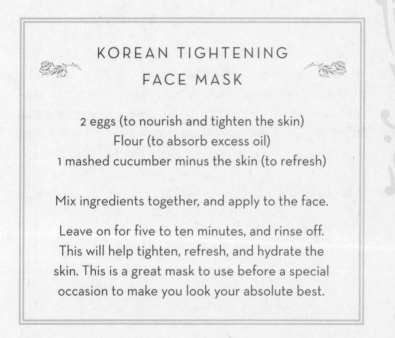

KOREAN TIGHTENING FACE MASK

2 eggs (to nourish and tighten the skin)
Flour (to absorb excess oil)
1 mashed cucumber minus the skin (to refresh)

Mix ingredients together, and apply to the face.

Leave on for five to ten minutes, and rinse off. This will help tighten, refresh, and hydrate the skin. This is a great mask to use before a special occasion to make you look your absolute best.

BRUSH AWAY THE DULLNESS

Dry brushing has been a secret of Japanese women for centuries. Starting your daily bathing routine with a quick sloughing of dead skin cells will ensure soft, smooth skin. Before stepping into your bath or shower, lightly massage your dry body in a circular motion using a bath brush. This method removes dead skin cells without getting rid of the protective oils and helps boost circulation and detoxify the body. Rinse away the dead cells as you step into the water, leaving touchable, softer skin.

Curing Your Cuticle Woes

I usually visit north India, closer to the Himalayan Mountains, in the winter months, when the weather is almost always cold and dry. Without fail, my cuticles will start splitting and cracking almost to the point of no return! I finally begged my cousins to show me what to do. Here is their secret: For dry cuticles, Indian women dip their nails in neem oil (available at any Indian grocery store), wrap their hands in cellophane under a hot towel, and after thirty minutes emerge with supple cuticles and strong nails.

Shalini's Beauty Tip

If you're trying to repair soft, brittle nails, or need to repair nails after getting your acrylics removed, applying this oil every night before bed will help to strengthen nails in no time! If you can't find neem oil, try almond oil.

SHINE ON!

Shiny hair is a definite fashion must in China! Take 1 teaspoon of rosemary oil and mix it with a cup of green tea. Pour it over your head as a final rinse for hair that really shines.

GET RID OF YOUR BAGGAGE!

For de-puffing puffy eyes, rose water is the trick for northern Indian beauties. Soak 2 cotton pads in rose water, and apply to each eye. Lay back and relax for five minutes. Remove and say good-bye to puffy eyes.

RELAXING YOU WITH YUZU

Add peeled strips of *yuzu,* the unique, exotic Japanese citrus fruit, to the bathwater when you fill the tub. As you bathe, the aromas will have a calming effect on the senses. If you can't find *yuzu,* try grapefruit, oranges, or tangerines.

SPICE THINGS UP!

Togarashi, or Japanese red chili peppers, can be used to warm up your feet and stimulate circulation, which means prettier pedi toes. Fill a bowl or foot bath with hot water, and add a few dried red chili peppers. Sit and soak your feet in the water for about ten minutes. Pat dry with a towel, and moisturize.

Be a (Nuka) *Bag Lady!*

Enjoy a luxurious skin-smoothing experience with *nuka* (Japanese rice bran) bath bags. Moisten the small muslin bag, and use it to rub your wet skin. This will leave your skin feeling soft and smooth. *Nuka* can also be used on the face instead of soap.

ASIAN DIET TIPS

Traditionally very healthy cultures, Asian countries such as China, Japan, and Thailand offer dishes full of fish, rice, legumes, and soy. Indian foods are aromatic and rich with spices and natural flavorings. Based mainly on a vegetarian diet, the Indian meal is balanced delicately with all food groups. Exotic dishes and curries are prepared with spices that are added carefully to each dish to maintain balance in digestion and overall health. Never discount the health benefits of green and black teas, which accompany most meals.

If you've ever traveled through Asia, you can't help but notice how fit the women are. Here are a few of Asia's best tips for staying healthy, slim, and fabulous!

Lemon Aid to the Rescue

Start your morning with a glass of warm water with the juice of half a lemon. In India, all my cousins and their friends begin their day with this secret—an instant detox that speeds up their metabolism.

WARM AND COLD DON'T MIX

Drink warm liquids with all your meals. Ice-cold liquids are said to interfere with digestion.

BREATHE AWAY STRESS

Start your day with yoga. Daily yoga breathing is said to be the breath of life. Breathing exercises that are based on breathing diaphragmatically are said to give your skin a glow that is unmatched by any store-bought product.

SUPERSIZE YOUR VEGGIES

Eat a diet that is full of leafy, green vegetables. In countries like Korea and throughout Southeast Asia, the everyday diet is full of dark, green, leafy vegetables that are rich in antioxidants and vitamins for healthy skin and body!

PROCESSED WHAT?

Eat fresh foods. Stay away from processed foods for optimum living. My relatives shop daily for fresh ingredients for each meal.

LISTEN TO YOUR BODY

Practice portion control. Eat small meals throughout the day, and stop when you feel full. I do this every time I go to Asia, and somehow manage to lose weight. It's the best way to diet because it's not deprivation, which can lead to binge eating. You can eat what you want—just in moderation!

OOLONG YOUR BODY

On my last trip to San Francisco, I stopped by for a tea ceremony at DynasTEA shop. My friend May, who owns the shop, gave me the lowdown on which teas do what. When I asked for her favorite for glowing skin, she looked at me and said, "White tea, of course!" Naturally, I also had to know which tea is good for keeping you slim. She promptly brought me a cup of hot oolong tea. So there you have it—I've been drinking oolong ever since!

SHALINI'S ASIAN MAKEUP TIPS

One thing I noticed throughout Thailand was how the women there love wearing bright eye shadow colors. If they were wearing a bright teal silk jacket, they coordinated their eye shadow to match. Don't be afraid to spice up your makeup routine with some bold, beautiful colors! If you want to experiment but are color shy, opt for textures that are sheer or cream-based. That way you will brighten up your look without looking overdone! If you are still wary of color, try an eyeliner pencil in your favorite color. It's a great way to play up your eyes in an instant, without being overbearing!

Here are a few tips I use on my celebrity clients:

• Use navy blue mascara instead of black to brighten the whites of your eyes.

• Stay away from using colors that match your eye color. Lining green eyes with a green eyeliner is like golfing with a green golf ball—no contrast! Stick with colors that contrast and complement your eye color. Here are few complementary color matches that will make your eyes the prize:
  • For green eyes use plums, violets, red-based browns, peaches, and oranges.
  • For blue eyes use burgundy-based browns, slate grays, lilacs, and colors with cooler undertones.
  • For brown eyes use any color other than colors with gray undertones, which can make you look dull and tired.
  • For hazel eyes use plums, plum-based browns, rich khakis, and anything with a warm orange undertone.

One feature I absolutely love about Japanese women is their rosy glow. Every time I travel to Japan I can't help but notice how fabulous their cheeks look. So for a change, play up your cheeks for a romantic, flushed look. Keep your eyes and lips soft, and apply a bright pink or peach blush just to the apples of the cheeks. You'll look instantly healthy and youthful!

An Instant Eyelift—Sans Surgery!

If you're looking for an instant eyelift without going under the knife, do I have a tip for you! I found one of the best beauty secrets on my last trip to Asia. I was sitting next to a beautiful woman on my flight, and as we were getting closer to landing she pulled out these ultracool eye tapes. Of course I had to know all about them. She explained that Asian women love to use the tape to make their eyes look bigger. By applying the eye tapes to their lids, they create the illusion of a crease by lifting the eye. As soon as I landed, I ran to the nearest beauty store to pick a few up for myself. I figured, if it works to create a crease, why wouldn't it work to lift saggy lids? Sure enough, I experimented and played and instantly lifted my lids. It was plastic surgery without the knife! If you have sagging lids, look down, pull the lid taut, and apply the tape directly to the crease. Your instant eyelift will make you look ten years younger.

The tapes are super sheer, so you can wear them with or without makeup. I thought they were so fantastic that I had to share them with everyone!

Create a Come-Hither Gaze

If it's the sultry mystique of Indian women that you desire, remember that it's all about the eyes. Make sure you start with perfectly groomed eyebrows. Threading is a great way to start! Then follow with a rich, colored eyeliner. Try a cake liner instead of a pencil if you want longer wear. For daytime, opt for a rich brown or deep navy. Black looks better in the evening, as it can tend to look too harsh in the daytime. Try the Global Goddess BoHo Exotic Eyes Kit.

3

A Beauty Safari Through Africa

Our next adventure is an exotic African beauty safari. From the great pyramids of Egypt over Tanzania's Serengeti to the stunning tropical beaches of Mombasa, this travel is sure to open your mind and bring you back into Mother Nature's arms. Africa is a destination full of time-honored traditions, rich cultures, and hidden treasures waiting to be discovered.

What a huge treasure it is! Africa is the second largest of the Earth's seven continents (Asia wins that title) and covers 23 percent of the world's total land area. It contains 13 percent of the world's population.

With such an expanse of land, it's no wonder it's a land of great diversity. If you were to trek across the continent, you would pass through lush, green forests and wander vast, grassy plains. You would cross barren deserts, climb tall mountains, and traverse some of the mightiest rivers on Earth.

DESTINATIONS

Egypt, Eritrea, Ethiopia, Gambia, Kenya, Morocco, Mozambique, South Africa, Sudan, Zimbabwe, and more

LOCAL BEAUTIES

Throughout Africa women are known for their beautiful bone structure and exquisite facial features. High cheekbones, full lips, and a lean physique make these women celebrated by many. With a long history of tribal culture, these women also hold a unique link to mysteries of beauty. From the hidden beauty secrets of Cleopatra to the tribal rituals of the Masai women of Kenya, these women look to the earth for raw, organic ways to make themselves beautiful.

A TASTE OF THE REGION

When you think of African cuisine, think traditional fruits and vegetables, exotic game, and fish from surrounding waters—all dishes are composed of a lovely mélange of cultures, colonies, trade routes, and history. Staple foods include *ugali* (a thick cornmeal mush), rice, bread, *chapati* (fried paste of wheat powder), beef, chicken, goat, and fish such as tilapia (a freshwater fish rich in omega-3). Cassava root is another staple of the African diet. Otherwise known as yucca root, the cassava is served much like a potato side dish. I remember growing up eating cassava root, boiled or roasted with a twist of lemon and an array of exotic spices sprinkled on top.

South Africa also has much of the French and British influences in its dishes, while Portuguese-influenced spices flavor foods in Mozambique and Angola. The most well-known alcoholic drink that has quenched the lips of thirsty Ethiopians for centuries is honey wine, or *tej.* With a little help from the earliest domesticated creatures (bees!), this wine is a slightly acquired taste, comparable to mead. Ethiopia also lays claim to the first cup of coffee. Java lovers welcome the Ethiopian coffee ceremony, which includes lighting incense, passing around the beans for the guest's approval, and their immediate roasting (of course, I mean the beans).

In Eritrea, a country that borders Ethiopia and Sudan, sleepy-eyed early risers start their morning with a pick-me-up called *silsi,* a peppery fried tomato and onion sauce usually served for breakfast. Travelers in the western lowland towns munch on an afternoon treat of *legamat* (deep-fried dough) from vendors. Other typical dishes through the region: *tsebhi,* a fiery sauce; *capretto,* roasted goat; and the vegetarian delight of *nai tsom.*

WEATHER REPORT

Africa straddles the equator, and most of its area lies within the tropics. To the west, the Atlantic Ocean; to the east, the Indian Ocean and Red Sea; and to the north, the Mediterranean Sea. In the northeastern corner of the continent, Africa is connected to Asia by the Sinai Peninsula. The climate ranges from the year-round heat and humidity of equatorial regions to the dryness of the world's largest desert (the Sahara) to mountaintop conditions cold enough to support blizzards.

BEAUTY SECRETS OF AFRICA

Many of my fondest childhood memories have to do with traveling to Africa. My mother was born in Kibigori, Kenya, and growing up we would go there every few years to visit my grandparents. We'd stay for months at a time. We made stops along the way in Egypt (I got the chicken pox there—talk about a beauty disaster!), Asia, and Europe. It was always an adventure, to say the least. My grandfather would set up exotic safaris in Kenya to coincide with the migration of animals like elephants, wildebeests, zebras, giraffes, and hippos across the Tanzanian border. It was breathtaking to be so close to nature and within arm's reach of thousands of animals.

During those visits I remember how mesmerized I was with the unique beauty of African women. Whether it was the mystique of the Egyptian women, the cosmopolitan fashion sense of the women of South Africa, or the decorated necklines of the women of the Masai tribe, they were unlike anything I had ever seen before.

A VEGGIE A DAY KEEPS DRYNESS AWAY

I recently worked with beautiful makeup artist Jacqueline Mgido. Noticing her stunning skin and sing-song accent, I was immediately taken with her and went hunting for her beauty secrets. Discovering that Jacqueline was from Zimbabwe, I had her give me the dish on the beauty secrets from her homeland.

She told me that because it can get so hot during the year, women in Zimbabwe are very careful to hydrate and protect their skin. Try this exotic vegetable mask to hydrate your dry skin:

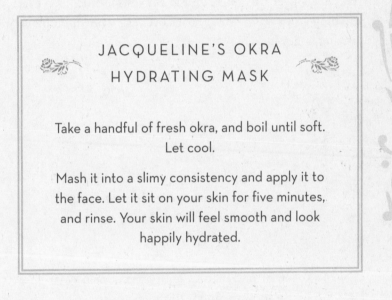

JACQUELINE'S OKRA HYDRATING MASK

Take a handful of fresh okra, and boil until soft. Let cool.

Mash it into a slimy consistency and apply it to the face. Let it sit on your skin for five minutes, and rinse. Your skin will feel smooth and look happily hydrated.

KOHL FOR DRAMA

Originally created to protect women's eyes from the blazing Middle Eastern sun, as well as shield them from diseases and impurities, *kajal* or kohl is used by today's African women for beauty. A thin line of this dark powder (brought to liquid form with a little water) along the eyes for day wear, a thicker, blurrier line for dramatic nighttime eyes.

A Sweet Hair Treat

A South African hair treat, this hair mask really gives your hair body and shine while helping with split ends. To get rid of the goo, give your hair a good lather, rinse, and repeat. If you have longer hair, increase the amounts a little. Don't let anything go to waste—use the leftover egg white for a moisturizing honey facial!

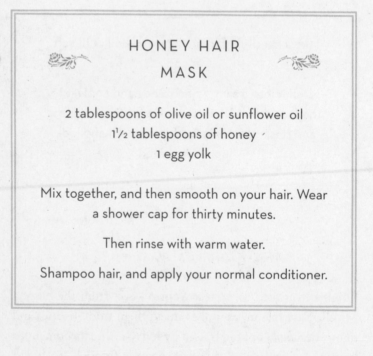

HONEY HAIR
MASK

2 tablespoons of olive oil or sunflower oil
1½ tablespoons of honey
1 egg yolk

Mix together, and then smooth on your hair. Wear a shower cap for thirty minutes.

Then rinse with warm water.

Shampoo hair, and apply your normal conditioner.

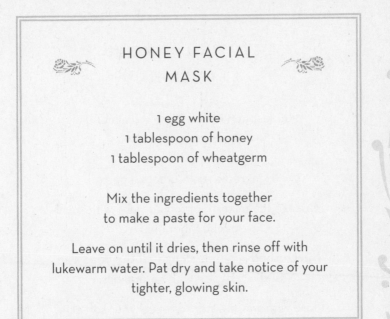

HONEY FACIAL MASK

1 egg white
1 tablespoon of honey
1 tablespoon of wheatgerm

Mix the ingredients together
to make a paste for your face.

Leave on until it dries, then rinse off with
lukewarm water. Pat dry and take notice of your
tighter, glowing skin.

SOFTEN DRY, BRITTLE HAIR

Egg and avocado is a popular African treatment for making hair soft. If you've ever been to Africa, then you know how large the avocados grow there! Take one soft avocado, and mush it up into a paste. Add an entire egg, and beat it until creamy. Rub the mixture over the hair and scalp, and wrap in plastic. It can be tough to wash out, but it's so worth the effort! Have some leftovers? The paste also makes a nice reviving face mask. That's double-duty beauty!

EGYPTIAN ALMOND EXFOLIANT

1 tablespoon of finely ground almonds
2 teaspoons of milk

Mix ingredients to create a paste.

Massage the mixture onto your face with small circular motions.

The crushed almonds slough off the dead skin and moisturize with natural oils.

Rinse with warm water to reveal your soft skin.

Shalini's Beauty Tip

Learn from the Egyptians. They know the trick to successful skin is hydration during exfoliation. One beauty blunder I often see is over-exfoliation. A lot of men and women—especially those with oily skin—feel the need to exfoliate with a heavy scrub. They forget that when one exfoliates, one must hydrate in order to avoid drying out the skin and causing unnecessary flaking and redness. Always follow your exfoliation with a moisturizer.

SKIN FIRMING WITH SAUSAGES?

Not actual tasty pork products, the fruits of the west African kigelia tree grown across sub-Saharan Africa hang from the branches and resemble huge sausages. What this fruit holds is magic—flavanoids and phytosterol saponosides that have long been recognized for their skin-firming abilities. Many generations of African healers have made skin-soothing creams from this tree's roots, bark, and fruits.

"BEN" THERE, DONE THAT

In a dry land of sandstorms and sun, ancient Egyptians relied on *behen* (or *ben*) oil to combat dry, aging skin. This pleasingly fragrant oil is derived from the nuts of the moringa or horseradish tree, also known as the "purifying tree." Just a few drops will yield a healthier and smoother complexion. This ancient oil is still available today, but to find it you may have to do research online or look for products that contain the oil, like the Clarins One Step Facial Cleanser.

SHEA BUTTER—A SECRET WEAPON

Shea butter is the perfect way to say you're sorry to your heat-damaged or overprocessed hair. It's a common ingredient in many moisturizers, and natural forms of it are as close as your local natural health food and drugstore. The women of Ghana have been using rich shea butter as a moisturizer and great humectant for conditioning hair, taming the frizzies by smoothing the hair cuticles, and giving it a special shine. After picking the fruit of the plentiful karite trees found on the west coast of Africa, these women remove the nuts, boil them, and leave them to dry in the sun. They are then roasted and crushed, then heated until the "butter" is released. The Global Goddess Shine Coconut Amla Revitalizing Hair Treatment includes rich shea butter for ultrasoft hair.

Ring Around the Rosy

Rosy cheeks give off a glow that says, "I'm healthy and happy!" Middle Eastern women take no exception to this face fact—they dab on a red stain called *akkar*, which is sold in clay pots throughout the marketplace. No messy applicator needed—women just wet their fingers, dip them in the pot, and rub the potion onto their lips and cheeks for instant color.

Shalini's Beauty Tip

Give yourself an instant healthy glow by wearing blush colors with pink and/or peach undertones— the brighter, the better. The trick to pulling off these bright colors is opting for textures that are sheer. Apply blush only to the apples of the cheeks—flash a big smile in the mirror, then dust the blush in a circular motion to the apples of the cheeks.

Dandruff Control

Any Ethiopian woman will whisper that the secret to soft, silky hair and a dandruff-free scalp is in *parfin* oil, or as we know it, paraffin oil, available at any Ethiopian food store and at most restaurants. These gals use this oil on their scalps at least once a week as a pre-wash scalp treatment. They advise leaving it in for at least thirty minutes prior to shampooing. Their mantra? The longer in the hair, the better!

Funny Name, Amazing Oil Control

A quick visit to the Moroccan marketplace, where a natural powdered conditioner called *rhassoul* is sold in large baskets, brings you one step closer to livelier hair. *Rhassoul* is mixed with water to form a paste, then applied to the hair and rinsed out after an hour. Moroccan women look to *rhassoul* clay, an ancient clay found in the Atlas Mountains of Morocco, to help with oil control and to give their hair incredible volume. You can find *rhassoul* products online or at any African grocery store.

Egyptian Spritzer

In ancient times, the Egyptians cornered the market on perfumes and fragrances. Lovely fragrances made from beautifully scented flowers from the Nile River Valley were available to anyone, but perfume itself was an expensive luxury item created only for the elite and was stored in lovely alabaster containers. To create the subtle scents of ancient Egypt, add a few drops of essential oils (like cinnamon, frankincense, lemongrass, myrrh, and rose) to a teaspoon of a bland vegetable oil (like sweet almond or grapeseed). Dab on your pulse points, and enjoy a warm rush of scent.

Shalini's Beauty Tip

A little heavy-handed with the perfume? Take a cotton ball soaked in rubbing alcohol, and blot the area on which you have sprayed or dabbed too much scent.

SHINE BRIGHT WITH STEAM

On a recent trip, I met a woman named Makda who had the most amazing bone structure. Her cheekbones were to die for, and her skin . . . well, let's just say there was not a blemish in sight. She was exotic and unique, to say the least. The mystique of her features was so captivating, it had me curious. She told me she was from Eritrea, so I had to know what she did to get and keep her flawless skin. She explained that that it was common practice in Eritrea for women to use steam to make their skin shine—especially before any important occasion, like their weddings. They cover their faces and bodies with a blanket, and allow the steam to hydrate the skin to bring back their natural glow. That sounded right to me!

After all, for years, almost every spa in the world has been clued in to the benefits of steam. It helps to boost circulation and rid the skin of toxins. Just a word of caution: Steam isn't for everybody. Keep your time in the steam room to a minimum, and avoid full-body steam if you are pregnant.

The Serum of Youth

One of the oldest medicinal plants, fenugreek's earliest recorded use dates back to the ancient Egyptians. Rumor has it there were even a few fenugreek seeds found in King Tut's tomb! For cosmetic purposes, fenugreek seeds have a reputation as a skin softener and are often a component of facial masks that soothe irritated skin.

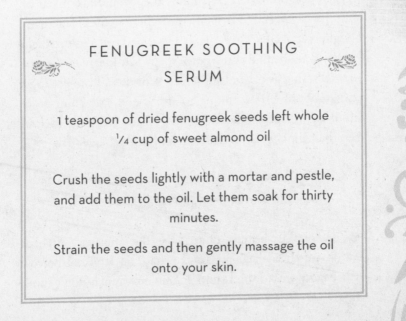

FENUGREEK SOOTHING SERUM

1 teaspoon of dried fenugreek seeds left whole
¼ cup of sweet almond oil

Crush the seeds lightly with a mortar and pestle, and add them to the oil. Let them soak for thirty minutes.

Strain the seeds and then gently massage the oil onto your skin.

FENUGREEK FOR BRIGHTER SKIN

Looks like the Ethiopians have a trick or two up their sleeves, as well, when it comes to fenugreek! They use it as a skin brightener and lightener. They make a face mask using fenugreek seeds and honey. Mix 2 tablespoons of honey with a handful of crushed fenugreek seeds in a bowl. Apply liberally to the face and neck, and relax for ten to fifteen minutes (although these gals tell me there's no rush when it comes to pampering!). Wash off and glow!

LYE DOWN FOR SUNSCREEN

One fun and unique secret I learned in Kenya came from watching the employees that worked for my grandfather. Every day before leaving for home, they would take a bar of white lye soap and rub it all over their bodies. I actually thought it looked a little silly at the time until I asked them the reasoning behind this strange soapy act. I learned that the lye soap acting as natural sunscreen kept them from getting a nasty sunburn. After talking to my friend Jacqueline from Zimbabwe, it seems like these beauties use the same trick to keep their skin cool, moisturized, and sun damage–free.

BEAUTY FROM THE BEAST

No one holds beauty quite like the majestic Arabian stallion—its head held high and proud. So why not borrow their beauty tips! Sound funny? Arabian women don't think so. Those who want smooth, shiny hair turn to the tricks of keeping these horses' gorgeous manes flowing—a hair rinse made from the brewed peel of the quince fruit.

GEE, I CAN'T BELIEVE BUTTER MADE YOUR HAIR SO SOFT

In the African Horn region, women swear by the qualities of naturally made butter to provide nutrients and moisture for the hair and scalp. Although a little pungent, it's very effective when smeared on generously and left under hot towels! The gals in Ethiopia tell me that as the butter melts, it also makes a great facial moisturizer!

OLIVE OIL TO THE RESCUE . . . AGAIN

Pure olive oil is often used as a good all-round treatment for the hair and scalp. It can be left on overnight or for several hours. In fact, my friend Jacqueline explained to me how the weather in Zimbabwe is one of the biggest beauty challenges its women face. Because of the heat, women keep their hair in braids to avoid knots and nasty tangles. They also use olive oil in their hair two to three times a week to keep it soft and tangle-free.

NATURE'S OWN MOISTURIZER

The quintessential ancient beauty, Cleopatra relied on the sweetness of honey to hydrate her bronzed skin. A thin layer applied to the face creates a watertight film and permits the skin to re-hydrate. Leave on for ten minutes, and then rinse with warm water, giving the skin enough time to replenish the moisture. Note: It may be a little sticky and take some work to rinse off, but it will be more than worth the effort!

EGYPTIAN MILK BATH

Cleopatra was also known for her soft-as-silk skin. Her secret? A luxurious milk bath. The lactic acid gently exfoliates the skin as it softens it. Milk baths are a great treatment for rough, dry, or sensitive skin. Don't feel like lugging a gallon of milk to your tub? Add 2 cups of powdered milk into your bathwater, and take advantage of this Egyptian beauty's know-how.

NEED A BREATH MINT?

In Zimbabwe, women reach for the leaves of a fresh mint plant to brush their teeth and freshen their breath. Not a bad idea!

Shalini's Beauty Tip

Should you find yourself in need of a quick breath freshener after a meal and there's no mint in sight, munch on the parsley garnish from your plate. Parsley is known to help with bad breath.

DIET TIPS FROM AFRICA

Take the Time to Eat

African women tell me the secret to keeping their figures in check is taking time to eat their meals. Not rushing to finish allows these gals to listen to their bodies (not to mention their dinner companions' conversation) and avoid overeating.

Go Nuts!

For a healthy diet, consider going nuts! In the African nation of Gambia, health-conscious diners feast on many delicious meals that have peanuts as the main ingredient, such as the nation's traditional favorite dish, tomato and peanut stew. While we consider them fattening, nuts of all shapes and sizes can replace meat or poultry as a great source of protein for any meal. Not only do the Gambians not have weight problems, but they also have the lowest international incidence of all types of cancer, according to the National Cancer Institute.

Get Up and Go!

These African gals say walking is not only a way of life but also a great way to keep their lean physiques. Walking around town is an easy path to a tight butt and strong, toned legs!

EAT TO LIVE

African women come from the school of "eat to live," not "live to eat." They look to basic staples to sustain their energy instead of using food as a source of comfort. No ice cream with a big spoon for them at the end of a stressful day.

TEA TO START

Tea is a major staple of the African diet. The women of Zimbabwe start their days off with a cup of hot tea with lemon. This is their secret to cleansing their system and keeping their metabolism working 'round the clock.

CARB-FREE? WHAT'S THAT?

In stark contrast to the carb-free diet being pushed in America, the African diet is actually high in starch, with much of the meal based around carbs. Do these gals worry? No way. When asked, they will quickly point out their daily walking (miles and miles fueled by the energy of the carbs) is what gives them amazing hourglass figures.

SHALINI'S AFRICAN MAKEUP TIPS

One fantastic feature common to just about every African woman I have met is sky-high cheekbones. Not all of us are blessed with this fabulous facial feature. But there's no need to worry. Here are a few tips for achieving jaw-dropping, sexy cheeks.

The Perfect Tools for the Job

As with any project, the tools you have determine how easy your job will be. When it comes to blush and sculpting your face, it's imperative to have the right brushes. If you're using a big powder brush and wondering why you're not getting sculpted cheeks, it's time to put that brush down! Look for brushes cut in a rounder, narrower shape, or angular ones that are cut to contour the cheek. You might also want to opt for brushes that have really soft bristles. Remember, the softer the bristles, the softer and more user-friendly the makeup application.

Shalini's Beauty Tips

Every Global Goddess should have the right tool kit in her makeup drawer. Remember, the right tools equal less makeup and a more flawless application. Here's what you need:

Blush brush

Crease eye shadow brush

Synthetic angled brow/ liner brush

Lip brush

Tweezers

Powder puff

Blending eye shadow brush

Synthetic concealer brush

Eyelash curler

Makeup sponge

When traveling, pack lightly and take only the essentials, meaning the brushes you use most. Try the Global Goddess Mini Jet Setter Tool Case for a mini version of all the necessary tools.

Two Are Better Than One

When it comes to defining your cheekbones, two colors are always better than one. One dark color can make you fall into that '80s blush faux pas—one long stripe of blush.

Start with a warm taupe shade or bronzer, and apply it along your cheekbones, brushing downward from your ear to two fingers' distance from your nose. Then apply a pop of color on the apples of your cheeks.

Shalini's Beauty Tip

Heavy-handed with the blush? Apply a loose powder over excess blush to soften your mistake.

AIM HIGH WITH PIGMENT

One common beauty challenge I heard about from the women of Africa was the inability to find colors that match their skin tone or colors that even show up on their darker complexion.

The solution? Makeup that is high in pigment or specifically formulated for women of color. Most professional makeup artists tend to use higher pigment levels in their products. You can tell if a color is high in pigment by swiping it on the back of your hand. If the color disappears or turns gray, then you know that the pigment level is low. If the color stays true to the color in the compact, then you know it is higher in pigment.

Finding foundation to match your skin tone can also be a challenge if you are a woman of color. I recommend custom blending your own foundation if you have a tough-to-match skin tone. Most professional makeup artists' lines will make pure pigments that are sold individually, in addition to the base cream. Find a foundation color that matches your skin tone closely (Global Goddess Complexion Perfection Duo is formulated to work with hard-to-match skin tones), and then add a few drops of the appropriate pigment. Depending on your undertones, you may need to add more red to warm it up or more dark brown to deepen the color. Either way, custom blending your foundation means that you'll be able to change color throughout the seasons (meaning if you get a tan in the summer, you can adjust your color by making it darker, and vice versa for winter skin tones).

4

The Good Old
U.S. of A.

Welcome home! Look around you—there are beauties right in your own backyard! After our whirlwind travels across the seas to the Ivory Coast, the Great Wall of China, and through the deserts of Rajasthan, let's not forget the beauty of the good old U.S. of A. These fifty states of ours offer beauty enthusiasts a unique blending of cultures and international influences. After all, the United States is the melting pot of the world! With the Pacific Ocean to west, the Atlantic to the east, and bordered to the north and south by Canada and Mexico, respectively, the U.S. is a source of many beauty traditions and trends. Our journey through the States will show us the reasons why everyone goes crazy for California avocados; why women in Hawaii know that as delicious as macadamia nuts are, they're also the secret to smooth, glowing skin; and down south, some sweet peaches may be exactly what the dermatologist ordered. This will be the best beauty road trip you've ever been on!

DESTINATIONS

Just one country, but fifty fabulous states, from the East Coast to the West Coast, right down the middle, and straight over to Puerto Rico

LOCAL BEAUTIES

As cultures blend in the U.S. creating sensational mixed skin tones, American women are the epitome of multicultural beauty. Depending on where they live or what job they hold, women in the U.S. have an eclectic sense of style and beauty. From the fresh-faced Texan girl next door to the sultry, sexy Manhattan siren, American women dominate beauty across the board, follow trends, and know how to play up their best features.

TASTE OF THE REGION

Depending on where you call home within the borders of the U.S., your diet will vary. From a heavy Mexican influence in California, to some good old jambalaya in New Orleans, wherever you travel, you're bound to find a regional dish that showcases its city's specialty. Food is in abundance, and variety is the spice of life. With some of the best dishes being a fusion of east and west, these American women are inundated with delicious temptations. That being said, women in America are body conscious as well as health conscious, watching what they eat and when they eat it. They know to indulge without overindulging. And no snacking after 7 P.M., a savvy dieter's no-no.

WEATHER REPORT

From the Pacific Ocean to the west, to the Atlantic to the east, the weather in the U.S. varies regionally. Sunny California is a favorite for surfers to hit the waves, with a temperate temp of 68 degrees almost year-round greeting these SoCal water lovers. Moving up the coastline, Oregon and Seattle are a little cooler; here, rain is usually the name of the game. Moving east through the hot Vegas desert, the conditions become dry and the climate sizzles as hot as the nightlife. If you're looking for snow, head through the Midwest and right up into the Northeast. Cold winters freeze snowbunnies from the Dakotas all the way to Vermont and Massachusetts. If it's the sultry heat you crave, jet on down to Miami for some tropical heat. Or stay on the West Coast with a jaunt to Hawaii, where tropical weather is just one of perks of life on the islands!

BEAUTY SECRETS FROM THE GOOD OLD U.S. OF A.

One of my favorite reasons for living in the U.S. is the exposure to diversity. There are so many subcultures within subcultures . . . and with them, generations of beauty secrets that have been passed down long family lines, from mother to daughter. When you walk into your favorite neighborhood spa, you can see this melting pot of cultures coming together for signature treatments. Culture is everywhere!

Go West, Young Woman

Midwest cowgirls have realized that the cream used on horses' hooves works wonders on their own nails and cuticles. For stronger, thicker nails, dab a little hoof cream (available on-line or at pet supply stores) onto your nails and nailbeds once a day. The rich emollient gelatin makes nails grow strong and softens skin.

Shalini's Beauty Tip

Have cracked heels? I learned this little trick from a celebrity I worked with. Hoof cream works great to heal cracked, dry skin. Just slather it on before bed, and wear a pair of cotton socks over your feet. Wake up in the morning with supersoft—not to mention pretty—sandal-ready feet.

Hawaii is one of my favorite vacation destinations. The warm tropical breezes, the aqua blue ocean, the yummy tropical cocktails . . . and so many fabulous beauty secrets! Here are a few of my favorites.

I'M GOING BANANAS!

Yes, you should have some bananas—that is, if you want the hydrated skin and fortified hair of Hawaiian beauties. Not only do bananas make great skin hydrators, but they also improve the health and natural elasticity of your hair. Bananas contain the same potassium that keeps your heart beating strong and wards off muscle cramps. The perfect concoction for the damage inflicted by processing treatments like coloring and straightening? Just mash a banana in a bowl, and slather away. Leave this delicious treat on your hair for fifteen minutes, and wash (and I mean *wash*) away!

GET KOOKY WITH KUKUI

Kukui nut oil, from a Hawaiian plant high in essential fatty acids that helps promote healthy skin, is great for strengthening the bond between the upper and lower nail plates. Aloha, more flexible nails! Just rub it in once a day. Kukui nut oil also can replenish hair's luster and elasticity. Don't be afraid to give yourself a well-deserved scalp massage with this nourishing oil!

GINGER FOR EVERY MARY ANN

Hawaiian ginger awapuhi is the perfect solution for hair that has lost its way. Originally brought to the islands by settlers, the large, bright flower contains a liquid with moisturizing lipids that condition hair and greatly improve its integrity, which means incredible body and shine. And the natural sudsy foam makes it a gentle, moisturizing cleanser for everything—skin, scalp, and hair.

Shalini's Beauty Tip

Can't find the natural ginger awapuhi flower? No sweat! There are plenty of hair products on the market that include this nourishing ingredient. Just check your local beauty supply store for hair products that contain awapuhi. I like Paul Mitchell's Awapuhi hair line and Nature's Gate Rainwater Awapuhi Shampoo.

SWEET, EXOTIC HAIR CARE

On a recent trip to Maui, I was introduced to the most intoxicating shampoo—a secret of Hawaiians. On a waterfall climb, my guide picked off the stem of a fresh ginger flower, a gorgeous pinkish red blossom. The flower was beautiful, but that's not all. He squeezed a clear, thick liquid with a beautiful scent from the cone of the plant and told me to rub it on my hair and skin as a hydrator. Not only was my skin and hair as soft as could be, the experience was priceless.

SCRUB AWAY THE HAWAIIAN WAY

Want to minimize dry, scaly skin? Rub on Hawaiian tur-binado sugar derived from the islands' lush sugarcane fields. A natural antiseptic and a mild hydroxy acid (a natural sub-stance used for centuries in skin rejuvenation), raw sugar makes an excellent exfoliant and also aids in hydration. It's also gentler than a salt scrub, because it dissolves quickly.

Shalini's Beauty Tip

Sensitive to the abrasive feel of salt? Raw sugar works as a great alternative and makes you smell as sweet as pie!

GEORGIA'S PEACHES AND CREAM

Let's head down to Georgia for some southern hospitality and flawless-looking skin. For a peaches-and-cream complexion, turn to the sweet Georgia peach! Mouthwatering peaches have been a centuries-long favorite of any wise southern beauty who has wanted a youthfully dewy complexion. These golden globes are rich sources of skin-renewing alpha-hydroxy fruit acids (which help to slough off dead skin cells), along with vitamins A and C (to nourish new ones). Peach juice unclogs pores, banishes blemishes, lightens age spots, and reduces wrinkles, giving skin a fresher appearance.

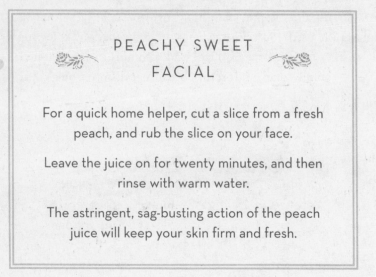

PEACHY SWEET FACIAL

For a quick home helper, cut a slice from a fresh peach, and rub the slice on your face.

Leave the juice on for twenty minutes, and then rinse with warm water.

The astringent, sag-busting action of the peach juice will keep your skin firm and fresh.

CALIFORNIA AVOCADOS—OUR SKIN'S BEST FRIEND!

As we age, time takes its toll on our bodies. Our skin begins to lose its moisture, making it drier and more dehydrated. Avocado masks are a great way to soften and soothe dry skin and give skin back its oomph. Rich in protein, vitamins, and fatty acids, is there anything this fruit doesn't offer? This little secret will be your best friend, should you ever suffer from scaly skin.

CALIFORNIA AVOCADO
SKIN HYDRATING MASK

1 California avocado (California avocados are the
best because of their higher oil content)
¼ cup of plain yogurt

Mash the avocado and add the yogurt to cool and
soothe the skin.

Brush the mask on your face and chill out for
about twenty minutes.

Rinse off and feel how soft and hydrated your
skin is.

SPEAKING OF AVOCADOS . . .

Avocado oil is great for the nails and cuticles. Because it's such a rich and nourishing oil, I always advise women who have just removed their acrylic nails, or who tend to have weak, brittle nails, to use avocado oil on their cuticles every night to strengthen their nail beds. It makes a huge difference! In fact, I'll never forget how traumatizing it was the few times I had to take off fake nail tips. Not only were my own nails short and stubby afterward, they were splitting right down the middle! It was so bad that I ran right back to the nail salon and had the tips reapplied. Bad idea. Avocado oil was my salvation and brought back my beautiful, healthy nails.

MORE SECRETS OF THE GREEN GLOBES

In Puerto Rico, a self-governing (and very independent-minded) territory of the U.S., women love to use avocados as a hair mask. You know the benefits (moisture, nourishment, protection from the sun), but here is the secret of ultrashiny, moisturized hair. My friend Hilda shares her mother's two favorite beauty recipes for glistening, soft hair.

HILDA'S AVOCADO HAIR MASK

1 avocado
1 cup of rosemary water (for brunettes only!)
(see the following recipe)

Take a ripe avocado, mash it up, and then push it through a sieve to get a smooth cream.

Massage it onto your hair and scalp; tie a scarf around your head, and leave it on for several hours.

Follow by washing your hair with a mild shampoo, and then use rosemary water for the final rinse.

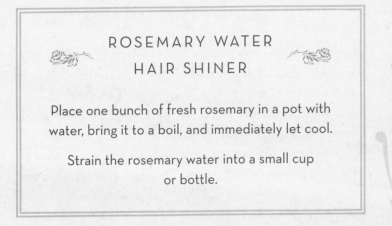

ROSEMARY WATER
HAIR SHINER

Place one bunch of fresh rosemary in a pot with
water, bring it to a boil, and immediately let cool.

Strain the rosemary water into a small cup
or bottle.

Shalini's Beauty Tip

Rosemary water works as a great hair shine for
brunettes. If you're a blonde, skip this step.

NATIVE AMERICAN ALL-AROUND BEAUTY FIX

It's pretty well known that cornmeal has been commonly
used by Native Americans, but what isn't well known is how
great it is for the skin. Simply make a paste with cornmeal
and water, and apply to the face or body, then rinse. It's a
gentle exfoliant for more youthful skin, a nourishing facial
mask, a great deodorizer for hands, and a super rub for prettier feet!

TEXAN BIG HAIR SECRET

There's nothing sexier than big, high-volume hair. But achieving it can be a quite the challenge if your hair is buried under tons of hairspray and product buildup. Take this tip from a Texan actress I used to work with in Hollywood. Coarse sea salt (a large, coarse, crystallized salt) mixed with a little shampoo works as a great exfoliating hair treatment. This secret mixture will remove product buildup, increase volume, and make your hair shine! I usually make a small container's worth and keep it in the shower for weekly doses. A great hush-hush tip if you've got a hot night out! If you don't have time to make some of your own, LUSH Cosmetics makes a great shampoo called Big.

Shalini's Beauty Tip

Curled lashes are the quickest way to make your eyes look bigger and brighter! Curl before applying mascara. For an extra wide eye, curl again after applying mascara, but be careful—pulling out eyelashes isn't sexy. Be gentle and take your time.

WIDE-EYED SECRET

Big, bright eyes are every girl's best friend. Here's a little tip I picked up on a photo shoot. For an instant eye opener, use the round end of a teaspoon at the base of your lashes. Gently push your lashes up and around the spoon.

SELF-TANNER BOO BOOS BEGONE!

Self-tanner gone awry? No worries! We all know how awful self-tanner looks when it dries on the wrong places on your hands, ankles, elbows, and all those other tricky areas. Here's a little secret I picked up from the gals in California: Use a cotton ball soaked in creamy cuticle remover. Apply on and around your ankles, hands, and feet to remove excess self-tanner. Now you're a bronze beauty with nothing to hide!

MOM MAY KNOW BEST

Growing up in California, I remember my mom was always using something from the refrigerator or pantry to soften her skin or help with her hair. One of her favorite instant hair masks that zaps away the dry frizzies is mayonnaise. Not only does it taste great on just about everything, but it also works as a great conditioner for dry hair. Take ½ to 1 cup of mayonnaise and apply it to dry hair. Give yourself a nice scalp massage and work it in through your hair. Leave it on for fifteen to twenty minutes before shampooing. For added benefits, wrap your hair in clear wrap, or apply a plastic grocery bag over your hair. The heat will increase the hydrating benefits of the mayonnaise.

OATMEAL—A NEW ENGLAND WINTER SKIN SOOTHER

With the winter winds swirling around them, New Englanders love a big bowl of piping-hot oatmeal to start their day, and a nice oatmeal bath to end it. Not only does this ingredient for a fiber-rich breakfast warm you up from the inside out, it also makes for a comforting bath to aid dry, itchy skin. Pour a cup of dry oatmeal into a piece of cheesecloth, tie into a ball, and plop it into a warm bath. This oatmeal "milk" is perfect for soothing the itchy scales of winter skin.

BRUSH AWAY CHAPPED LIPS

Take this tip from some models I worked with in Las Vegas. The desert heat and dry, arid conditions made keeping smooth lips a challenge for these gals. Follow their lead by gently brushing your lips with an old toothbrush with a small amount of moisturizer on it. Not only will you brush off any dead, dry skin, but you will also hydrate your lips!

Shalini's Beauty Tips

When exfoliating your lips, be it with an old toothbrush or a store-bought lip scrub, make sure to follow with a good moisturizing lip treatment. In fact, it's always good practice to apply a lip treatment every night before bed. Remember, sexy lips aren't chapped lips!

Vermont Moisture Secret

No one likes a wind-burned face! (We would rather have rosy cheeks from blushing at a compliment!) To avoid this wintertime woe, Vermont skiers smooth a thin layer of Vaseline all over their faces to combat windburn, frostbite, and dry skin. The petroleum jelly helps keep in moisture and warmth. Be sure to wash off once you're inside and warming up, so your pores won't clog.

An Orange a Day Keeps Dull Skin Away

Slough away dull skin with the sweet taste of oranges. Start off your day with some freshly squeezed orange juice (vitamin C for healthy skin), and save the rind. The girls in Florida use the citric acids in the orange rind to gently exfoliate dull skin and to add an instant luster to their skin. Try this mask to give your skin an instant glow!

CITRUS YOGURT MASK

1 orange
³/₄ cup of plain yogurt

Grate the rind of one orange and mix with yogurt.

Apply to skin (avoiding the eye area) and let sit for ten minutes.

Rinse and follow with a good moisturizer.

EASY, SEXY LOCKS

For show-stopping shiny locks, the girls in the South know what works best! Not only is baking soda a help in the kitchen, it also works great for getting rid of product buildup and styling goop. Add a little to the palm of your hand along with a dollop of shampoo, and wash away. You'll leave your shower with sexy, shiny hair. But be careful with this treatment—only clarify your hair once a week, or your gold will turn to straw.

BAKING SODA AGAINST BUILDUP

If you're like me and suffer from sensitive skin, especially in the wintertime, try this at-home scrub that will make your skin glow and keep the irritation at bay. Mix ¾ cup of baking soda with ¼ cup of water. Mix to a paste and use in a scrubbing motion on your face and body. You'll love this for the instant glow without the redness other harsh scrubs may leave behind.

EAST TO WEST SUN PROTECTION

Take the cues from thousands of skiers and beachgoers. Whether racing down the slopes in Colorado or lounging under an umbrella on the beaches of Key West, everyone knows to use sunscreen. Be extra careful near highly reflective surfaces such as sand and snow. Rub on a little sunscreen even if you're lounging underneath a beach umbrella. The sand can reflect 17 percent (and snow 80 percent!) of the sun's harmful rays.

Shalini's Beauty Tip

No matter what color your skin is or where you live, sunscreen is a beauty must-have. It's the secret to younger-looking skin because it protects your skin from the damaging rays that cause premature aging. It also helps prevent hyperpigmentation and sun spots.

BATTER UP FOR BEAUTY!

Nothing says America like baseball. Try those same sunflower seeds you see the boys of summer chomping on during the ninth inning as a gentle facial scrub. Grind 1 cup of sunflower seeds (hulled) in a coffee grinder until they're the consistency of finely grated Parmesan cheese. Mix the powder with a tablespoon of water, and rub gently on your face for a great exfoliation.

FLASH THAT HOLLYWOOD SMILE

In Hollywood, the secret to any superstar's success is a dazzling, white smile. Place a little baking soda in the palm of your hand, and add a small amount of hydrogen peroxide. Use this mixture to brush your teeth.

Shalini's Beauty Tip

A white smile is the easiest way to a more youthful look. Take ten years off your face by whitening your smile and avoiding dark lip colors like red, which can make your teeth look yellow.

DIET TIPS OF THE U.S.

Women of the U.S. love to stay current with the hottest diets and exercise plans. And media ideals can play a huge part in the success or failure of America's top diets. From cutting carbohydrates to eating a grapefruit after each meal, women of the U.S. are always looking for the next best diet tip or weight loss secret. They have twice the success in losing those unwanted pounds by teaming up nutrition with a good exercise plan. Strength training helps keep your metabolism steady all day, and yoga and Pilates help these gals with picture perfect posture. In other words, not only do the women here love their beauty secrets, but they also make dropping pounds and maintaining a consistent weight one of their lifestyle rituals.

Here are a few of my favorite tips I've picked up working in Hollywood over the years, seeing every possible way to lose weight!

A Little Vinegar for a Little Figure

One little secret I picked up on a photo shoot with swimsuit models was the great benefits of apple cider vinegar. I talked to these hard-bodied models and asked for their secrets to a slim figure, and they all swore by drinking 1 tablespoon of apple cider vinegar every morning before starting their day. Not only does this shot help boost their metabolism, but it also gives their skin a fantastic glow.

Shalini's Beauty Tip

If you're a wimpy girl like me and can't stand the taste of pure vinegar, try apple cider vinegar tablets. Available at any health food store, this kinder version gives you the same results without making you wrinkle your nose first thing in the morning.

TIME IS OF THE ESSENCE

The skinny minis of the U.S. keep their meals on schedule. They believe the secret to staying slim is to avoid eating after 7 P.M. Some models and actresses I've worked with told me that they lost up to ten pounds within the first month of incorporating this new eating schedule.

FLOAT AWAY

As with just about every country, women of the U.S. know the benefits of drinking water. Not only for great-looking skin, but also for a slimmer body. Drink eight to ten 8-ounce glasses of water daily. Another secret? Drink one 8-ounce glass before every meal. It'll fill you up, so you won't reach for that second helping.

Got Milk? Get Fit!

The latest health news has us on the watch for slimmer figures with milk. Just four glasses of the white stuff a day (skim or low fat, if you please) actually can help you lose weight. You can also accomplish this with plenty of low-fat cheese and yogurt in your daily diet. And with newer studies showing that calcium can significantly reduce the severity of PMS symptoms . . . well, sign me up!

More Is Better—Just in Smaller Portions

For maintaining a consistent weight, nutritionists in the U.S. recommend eating five mini meals a day. This helps keep blood sugar levels from dipping, which may cause you to overeat and can slow your metabolism.

Carb Less

To keep weight down, trendsetters in the U.S. avoid carbohydrates. The secret is avoiding all "white" foods, meaning refined carbohydrates such as white flour, sugar, and foods high in starch.

> *Shalini's Beauty Tip*
>
> Don't forget carbohydrates are a very important part of your diet. Don't discard carbs that are found in whole grains and fruits.

SHALINI'S U.S. MAKEUP TIPS

Women in the U.S. love to follow the latest trends in makeup and hair. From the runways in New York to the latest celeb secrets in Los Angeles, women here are always looking for the next best beauty secret. Here are some of my favorite makeup tips I've used for years on some of your favorite celebrities and TV shows.

JUST GLOW AWAY

Women in the U.S. and all over Hollywood love to have that dewy, golden glow. To achieve this look, start by adding a drop of luminizing lotion (available in most beauty product stores) to your foundation. Luminizing lotion has a touch of shimmer to it, which causes light to reflect off your face. For a radiant way to look healthy and face every day with style, try the Global Goddess Upgrade Complexion Face Primer with Licorice.

Drop Weight with Hilighting

Every girl loves the look of a slim, chiseled face. Here's a quick tip I learned in Hollywood for getting great-looking cheekbones, not to mention the look of instant weight loss! Take a hilight color in a white or light pink shade. Apply subtly below your cheekbones, above your cheekbones, and down the bridge of your nose. Opt for a crème hilighter for a more natural effect, and skip the heavy contour!

Control Unruly Brows

Every beauty buff knows that the secret to a finished look lies in perfecting the eyebrows. Keeping brows shaped and groomed allows you to wear less makeup by creating a perfect frame around your eyes. This can be trickier for some women. As we get older, or if we have coarse hair, our brows can get a little unruly. So skip the expensive brow gels and use a little flake-free hair gel or hairspray. Apply a small amount to your finger, and brush it in an upward motion through your eyebrow. You'll look more finished instantly!

Mix and Match

Any professional makeup artist knows the secret to her success is in using makeup creatively. Love your blush but wish it could be a lip color? Think your lip gloss would make the perfect blush? Then make it so! Mix a dab of your blush color with clear lip gloss and voilà—you've got beautifully blushing lips! Same goes for that ultradewy look we're seeing hot off the runways. Use a dab of clear lip gloss on your cheeks and eyelids to add an extra sparkle to your beauty routine.

Glow, Baby, Glow!

Love the look of a year-round tan? Follow this beauty tip of models from sea to shining sea. Mix a dab of self-tanner with your body lotion, and apply daily. You'll maintain a beautiful tan year round!

Make Your Own Lip Stain

We all love the days of summer and the great lip colors those popsicles leave on our lips. Make your own summer lip stain by taking your favorite flavor Jell-O Gelatin and adding a touch of water. Dab right onto your lips for stay-proof lip color in a pop!

5

The

Americas—A

World Apart

O ur exciting journey through the world of beauty continues with the fifth stamp on our passport, the Americas. Two continents mean a very large and culturally diverse area—full of hundreds of secrets waiting for us to uncover! From our neighbors to the north all the way down to those South American beauties, we'll make stops and gather beauty tips from women who have always known that beauty begins with nature and that taking care of themselves is just one part of their daily routine. With a laid-back approach to life, their secrets are simple yet effective. Our adventure will take us through Canada, where beauty and lifestyle have quite the French flair, south through Latin America, and then it's off to relaxing stops in the ultralush and tropical islands of the Caribbean. With such a culturally diverse area to explore, we'll discover that no matter our destination, beauty is top priority.

DESTINATIONS

Bahamas, Belize, Brazil, Canada, Cayman Islands, Chile, Dominican Republic, Jamaica, Mexico, and Venezuela, just to name a few

LOCAL BEAUTIES

In South American countries like Brazil and Venezuela, cellulite-free bodies and thick, wavy hair make these women some of the most envied and beautiful women in the world. Throughout the south and the tropics, gorgeous tanned skin inspires an international obsession, forcing cosmetic companies to design products for the bronzed island goddess in each of us.

A TASTE OF THE REGION

Foods throughout Canada, South America, and the islands of the Caribbean are very diverse and delicious, to say the least. In the tropics, fresh fruits are the staple of every diet and are often found in delicious chutneys and sauces. Food here is healthy and brings an explosion of flavor to your taste buds. The Mexican and Central American diet consists of three meals a day, with lunch being the heaviest. (Most meals are rich in meats, cheese, and beans.) Diets in Venezuela, for example, are balanced with the main dishes, consisting of a variety of soups, meat, salads, and baked and fried bananas.

When talking to my Venezuelan friend Marlin about the traditional diet, she told me, "Of course, it's all about the *arepa*." The Venezuelan *arepa* is one of those delicious treats that can be eaten as a snack or as a meal, depending on how hungry you are. It's a corn muffin, crisp on the outside and fluffy on the inside, and is usually stuffed with delicious fillings like mashed chicken, shredded beef, cheese, avocado, and plantains. For our friends to the north, in Canada, it's *oui* to the French influence of cheeses, breads, and game meats.

WEATHER REPORT

Not only are North and South America culturally diverse, but also the climate conditions range from one extreme to the other. Canada, our neighbor to the north, characterizes its climate conditions regionally. Parts of Canada fall close to the Arctic region with extreme cold and frigid weather conditions, while the western regions enjoy relatively mild and warmer conditions, thanks to the Pacific Ocean. South America moves into warmer tropical climate, with most of the area receiving a large amount of rain from the tropical rain forests. Don't be fooled, though—South America is very diverse, with regions as dry as the desert and as cold as ice in the Andes Mountains. Beyond the south and a quick trip over to the Caribbean, tropical weather is an everyday luxury for islanders who only battle bad weather seasonally with the hurricanes.

BEAUTY SECRETS OF THE AMERICAS

Mexican Bodyliscious

On a recent trip to Careyes, Mexico (a fabulous hidden get-away that sits right on the Pacific Ocean, about two and a half hours south of Puerto Vallarta), I couldn't help but notice how the women there really went back to the basics. Food was cooked fresh, there was an abundance of fruits and vegetables on every plate, and each woman I spoke with told me how much Mexican women pride themselves on taking care of their skin, hair, and body naturally. Seems like simplicity is definitely the way to go.

One woman named Rocio had many great beauty secrets to divulge. Of course I couldn't wait to hear what the women of Baja did to get such radiant, soft skin.

Pacific Ocean Body Scrub

For radiant, smooth skin, Mexican beauties start their morning showers by taking handfuls of coarse sea salt and rubbing it onto their bodies, letting it mix with the water. Keep a container of coarse sea salt in your shower, and apply it with a circular motion while your skin is still dry, before bathing, for maximum exfoliating benefits.

Wake Up with a Smoothie

Then it's on to a smoothie . . . a body smoothie! The women in Careyes love this summertime treat. Rev up your blender in the morning by mixing together yogurt, strawberries, avocado, honey, and bananas. Then apply this smoothie all over your body as an instant hydrating mask. Fifteen minutes is all you need to rid yourself of any dry skin.

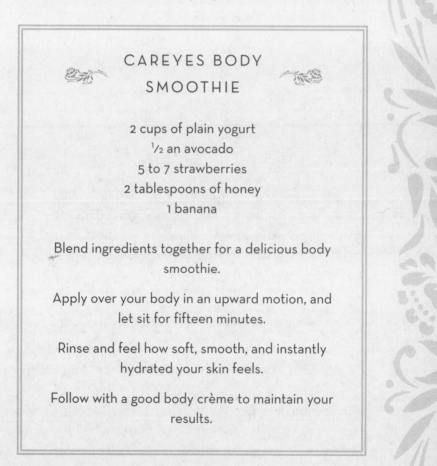

CAREYES BODY SMOOTHIE

2 cups of plain yogurt
½ an avocado
5 to 7 strawberries
2 tablespoons of honey
1 banana

Blend ingredients together for a delicious body smoothie.

Apply over your body in an upward motion, and let sit for fifteen minutes.

Rinse and feel how soft, smooth, and instantly hydrated your skin feels.

Follow with a good body crème to maintain your results.

Shalini's Beauty Tip

Fruits in this body smoothie are high in vitamin C,
which acts as a great antioxidant, protecting your
skin from free-radical damage. (Free radicals are
found in the environment in smoke or pollution
and can damage and age the skin prematurely.)
Using products that are high in antioxidants will
prevent premature skin damage and aging.

Shalini's Beauty Tip

The combo of the salt scrub and smoothie mask
will give your body that red carpet glow! Exfoliating
dead, dry skin allows your body to get the most out
of this moisturizing treatment.

BE SEXY LIKE A BRAZILIAN—TAKE IT ALL OFF!

Want to feel sexy like the Brazilians? Then take it all off!
These beauties go for the traditional Brazilian bikini wax for
hair removal. And we mean removal! Everything goes . . . ex-

cept for maybe a thin little strip. Not only does it make wearing bathing suits that much sexier, but it also gives these women a sense of confidence and a feeling of sexiness that they love!

Brazilian Tanning Secret

Brazilian women love to look their absolute best. That means keeping their waxing, manicures, and pedicures in tip-top condition. According to my friend Flavia, in the summer months these beauties munch on carrots and *beterraba* (beets) to maintain their infamous Brazilian tan.

Grape Expectations

Wake up your weary skin, draw out toxins, and stimulate circulation with a Chilean grape mask. Smash up a handful of grapes, and combine them with 1 teaspoon of white flour to form a thick paste. Pat onto your face, and let sit for twenty minutes before rinsing.

Fizzies Fighting Frizzies

The straight, sexy hair of a lovely from the Dominican Republic is enough to make anyone jealous. Her secret? Pouring on seltzer water after her final rinse in the shower. This fizzy, refreshing drink washes away the frizzies for straighter, shinier hair.

MILK YOUR MILK FOR ALL IT'S WORTH

Nothing says beauty like . . . milk film? It's true! Women in the Dominican Republic swear by the film on the top of boiled milk for softening their faces. Boil milk and let it sit. When it cools, it creates a soft film on the top. Peel off the film by dabbing your finger into it (it's sticky), mix gently with a little salt, and rub on your face. It's the perfect skin softener. Now on to your bath. . . .

DON'T GET BURNED

We've all done it . . . whether it's from a candle, a stove, or from a splash of hot grease while making dinner, we've all gotten burned. But don't let a scar be a permanent reminder. Women of the Dominican Republic dab tomato sauce on a burn to lower the chances of getting scarred. The lypocene in the tomato helps the skin heal faster. Now that's quick thinking!

BE A BABE WITH BABASSU

Found in certain areas of Brazil and other South American countries, the tall, wild-growing babassu palm trees offer beauty-conscious women a light, non-greasy skin moisturizer extracted from its nuts. Because babassu oil is a non-greasy moisturizer, it is especially good for oily skin. Smooth it on for hydrated skin. I also love to use it on my lips. Try the

Global Goddess Drench Hydrating Lip Spa, which contains babassu oil for extra hydrated lips.

PASSION RUNS DEEP

Looking at the not-so-pretty passion fruit, you'd never think that within its egg shape lies the secret to beautiful skin! It's my favorite fruit! Native to southern Brazil and Mexico, this exotic, dark purple fruit was named "passion" by Spanish missionaries, who saw symbols of the Crucifixion in the plant's flowers. Each passion fruit has as many as 250 magical seeds inside, waiting to deliver the ultimate in hydration! Once they are pressed, the seeds produce incredibly moisturizing and fragrant oil high in vitamins A and C. You can find many products that contain this easily absorbed oil online or at the Body Shop.

THE GREAT WHITE NORTH

Canada is one of those quick getaways that I always enjoy. Great shopping, fantastic food, and whenever I'm there, I bump into a new relative. (I seem to have hidden cousins hanging out in Canada.) The last time I visited Toronto, it was the middle of winter and freezing cold. Being a native Californian, that kind of cold was a shock to my system. It was also the first time I noticed my scalp flaking visibly. Of course a dry, flaky scalp was a huge beauty no-no, especially because I had meetings scheduled for the entire trip. So

what's a Cali girl to do? Here's a Canadian beauty secret that
I still use at home.

Canadian Cider to the Rescue

An apple a day to keep the itchy scalp away? It's true! Women
in Canada know the importance of a healthy scalp, so they
rinse their hair with apple cider after shampooing. The cider
restores hair's pH balance and soothes the dry scalp.

Warm Spots

If you love hot, tropical places like I do, then there's no question that the islands of the Caribbean are a definite must-see
destination. Book your ticket now because we're off to sip
some fruity cocktails and soak up some island sun. With its
turquoise waters and hot, humid climate, there are plenty of
exotic fruits and vegetables to tempt your tastebuds, skin, and
hair! These island beauties know exactly how to jump-start
their routines by keeping it natural.

Pineapple-a-Glow-Go

Golden, sweet pineapples are nature's great exfoliants. They
are everywhere in the tropics and have been used for centuries
for their smoothing effect on the skin. Their non-irritating
but hard-working fruit enzymes loosen dead skin cells, result-

ing in a soft, glowing, smooth complexion. For that special Caribbean glow, slice a ripe pineapple and massage the mashed fruit and juice onto your face. Let the sticky pulp dry completely for about ten minutes, and then rinse with warm water and pat dry. Just feel how much softer and more supple your skin is!

Shalini's Beauty Tip

If you suffer from sensitive skin or don't like to use abrasive face scrubs, products with natural active enzymes like pineapples are a great alternative. With pineapples, you'll get the same benefits of exfoliation without the grittiness that can cause dryness or irritation.

Go Bananas for Great Skin!

Caribbean beauties know how to protect their skin and treat a sunburn—all with a little help from Mother Nature. These beauties treat their skin with banana peels. After scooping out the banana fruit (for a smoothie, perhaps?), they rub the insides of the peels over their faces to soften and protect from the sun. They also use bananas on sunburned areas to help soothe irritated skin.

Yes, We Have Even More Bananas!

Following their Caribbean sisters, women in South America often use mashed bananas to help relieve dry skin and hair. A banana mask leaves a hydrated complexion after a quick rinse. You can also combine a few drops of almond oil with mashed bananas to relieve damaged hair. Massage into your hair and then allow it to work its wonders for about fifteen minutes. Because the oils and bananas are quite heavy moisturizers, rinse, shampoo, and condition as usual afterward.

"Guac" Away from Puffy Eyes

Guacamole is a fabulous side dish in Mexico and South America. It's made of mashed avocados, onions, cilantro, lemon, and chili spice, and is delicious, to say the least! In Mexico, the Aztec Indians have reveled in the many benefits of avocados for centuries. Known for its rich oils, avocados also work great as eye de-puffers. Just place one slice of fresh avocado under each eye, and lie back for fifteen to twenty minutes. Your puffiness will disappear!

Coconut for Safe Skin

Women in Belize use coconut oil directly on their skin to prevent sunburn. Not only does it create natural sunblock, but it also brings a dewy glow to the skin. Remember, these women use coconut oil as a day-to-day sunscreen and do not use it for sunbathing.

Shalini's Beauty Tip

Wherever you travel, make sure to wear a minimum of SPF 15 on your face and body to avoid premature aging and sun damage. If you're like me and have too many products to apply in the morning, remember to apply your sunscreen before your moisturizer. For added protection, double up your products: For example, opt for moisturizers with built-in sunscreens.

NOURISH YOUR SKIN WITH SEA WATER

Women in the Caribbean don't go any farther than right outside their doors for hydrated skin. Caribbean sea water contains minerals such as magnesium, calcium, bromide, and potassium that nourish skin and create a refreshed look. These beauties wash their faces with sea water for an unparalleled glow.

Shalini's Beauty Tip

For the same hydrating benefits, make your own face spray sans sea water with ½ cup distilled water and 2-3 drops of lavender oil. Pour into a spray bottle, and spritz on your face throughout the day. The water mixed with the essential oil is another secret you can have at home to hydrate your skin and bring about a lovely glow!

JAMAICAN ALOE—THE SECRET TO GREAT SKIN AND HAIR

I'll never forget the last time I was in Jamaica. The women were captivating with their flawless skin, incredible hair, and the most beautiful sing-song voices. In Jamaica, nourishing aloe vera plants are everywhere. Their tall light-green stalks seem to stick out from behind every building, home, and seaside village. Aloe has many uses, from steeping a cup of hot water to soothing troubled skin to food (its light-green pulp can be eaten straight from the plant)—Jamaican women turn to this succulent plant for almost anything.

You can also benefit from the healing properties of aloe by using aloe-based products on your body and hair. Easy to grow in your own home, aloe is exceptionally beneficial if you have been in the sun and need to treat sunburned or irritated skin. Just break off a stalk and squeeze the gooey nectar onto damaged skin for soothing relief.

A Slippery Ackee Bath

The national fruit, ackee, is more than just an ingredient for typical Jamaican meals. This slippery, slimy fruit is great for removing dead skin and controlling body odor. Jamaican women bathe with pieces of the fruit in their tub for a silky skin experience.

Fake Nails? Why Bother!

The women in the Dominican Republic know that beautiful nails mean beautiful-looking hands, and they know the secret to getting strong, hard, gorgeous nails without an expensive trip to the nail salon. These savvy women make their own nail strengthener at home by chopping up fresh garlic and adding it to clear nail polish. They let this little concoction sit for a week and then they apply it as a topcoat to their bare nails. Your nails may smell a little funny initially, but the result is hard to beat!

I'm Nutty for Shiny Hair

The women in the Cayman Islands use castor and nut oils in their hair for a high shine. Spend an evening at home and pamper yourself with a hot-oil scalp massage. Apply enough to coat your hair and scalp.

TAME PESKY FLY-AWAYS

Women in the Bahamas tame fly-aways with avocado oil. Rich in vitamins and proteins, this oil acts as a great hair moisturizer and will replenish dryness immediately. Add a few drops to your hands and rub them together. (The warmth allows the oil to spread more evenly.) Now rub your hands over your hair (don't rub the oil in, just stroke the top of your hair lightly) to show those fly-aways who's boss. We added avocado oil to the Global Goddess Shine Coconut Amla Revitalizing Hair Treatment. I know a few gals who love to rub a few drops over the hair for a frizz-free day! You can also find pure avocado oil at your local health food store.

EVEN MORE AVOCADOS . . .

Women in the Dominican Republic know that these gorgeous green fruits have more to offer than just a taste sensation. They use the mashed pulp to brighten their skin. The avocado's vitamin A–rich oils penetrate skin cells, leaving them silky smooth and nourished. And there's even more to this rich green mush than meets the eye. According to *The Encyclopedia of Chemical Technology,* avocado has the highest amount of sunscreen effectiveness when compared with other naturally derived oils.

TROPICAL ISLAND RADIANCE

For the fresh glow of an island beauty, cut open a ripe papaya, scoop out the pink fruit, and place the empty hull on your face. The leftover papain in the remaining pulp and skin peel is great for tackling rough skin and wrinkles. It's tough on wrinkles but gentle on sensitive skin.

Shalini's Beauty Tip

Feeling a little under the weather? Give your self a quick pick-me-up and healthy glow by adding a small amount of self-tanner to your moisturizer. It's one little trick for looking your absolute best!

A CARROT A DAY KEEPS THE TANNING SALON AWAY

The women down south have tanned skin that is envied by men and women around the world. But even they have little secrets to getting a deeper, more bronzed color.

We all love fruit juice in the morning, but for the women in Latin America, pineapple and carrot juice rank as their favorites, but not for obvious reasons. Two weeks before these women go to the beach, they begin to have a glass of fresh carrot juice every morning. They believe that the carrot juice gives their tans a spectacular bronze color.

Shalini's Beauty Tip

Carrots are high in vitamin C, help to detoxify the liver, and can protect the skin from melanoma, among many other benefits. Drinking carrot juice in large amounts, however, can cause a slight yellowing of the skin, which in turn can deepen a tan to a fabulous bronze color. Be warned: Too much of a good thing is just that—too much. Because of its high vitamin A content, you shouldn't drink carrot juice every day.

YOUR HAIR'S ON FIRE!

Linaza, otherwise known as flaxseed, mixed with hot water and used as a pre-rinse before shampooing, is a Latina secret for long shiny hair. These women also believe that *linaza* will help make their hair grow long, lush, and strong.

DIRTY LITTLE SECRET

Another little tip I learned while visiting Mexico involves the regular use of volcanic mud on the body. Mexican women have used this mud for ages to improve skin tone. The mud also acts as an anti-inflammatory and antiseptic, which in turn helps to draw out harmful toxins that might compromise the skin's beauty and health.

Shalini's Beauty Tip

Mud-based masks are an excellent way to detoxify the skin, tighten pores, and clarify your skin tone. If you have an uneven skin tone, masking with a clay will help even you out, leaving you with a more flawless complexion.

OILY HAIR MINT FIX

When your hair is too oily, turn to this quick-fix tip from the lovely Venezuelan ladies. Boil water with fresh mint leaves, and let cool. Remove the leaves and splash on this minty refresher as your final hair rinse in the shower. Not only is the scent uplifting, this toner will also help you tame the oils that can leave your hair limp.

Shalini's Beauty Tip

No time to wash your hair? Use baby powder to
give your hair an instant "shampoo." For a quick fix,
sprinkle a little powder on the roots of your hair.
Brush it through, and you're off with a fresh-looking
mane. For an added volume boost, aim your blow-
dryer at the roots while lifting your hair with your
fingers. The powder will also act as an
instant root lift!

OILY SKIN CURE-ALL

There's nothing worse than an oily shine. Mexican women
know that a few kitchen staples can help make that shine disappear. They apply a mixture of 1 tablespoon each of chopped
parsley (soothes with antiseptic qualities), milk (gets rid of impurities), and honey (takes care of hydration) to their faces.
After ten minutes and a quick rinse, the only thing that shines
is their beauty!

TOMATOES—A T-ZONE SECRET WEAPON

Tomatoes are plentiful in the South American diet, from sal-
sas to delicious sauces. And they are also a staple on the
beauty shelves of most beauty-conscious women. Not only

are these red fruits high in the cancer-fighting lypocene, they can also combat the T-zone blues. Venezuelan women apply mashed tomatoes directly to the T-zone and wash off after a few minutes. The naturally acidic tomato helps maintain the skin's pH balance while gently neutralizing oily conditions, refining enlarged pores, and providing soothing relief for troubled complexions.

Shalini's Beauty Tip

If you have dry or sensitive skin, skip the previous tomato tip, as it may cause some irritation.

MASH AWAY SPLIT ENDS

Dry hair and split ends are a common beauty challenge that many South American women face. Luckily, they can rely on the buttery, sweet avocados (a staple of the Latin American diet) to remedy the problem quickly.

Find a ripe avocado, and mash it up in a bowl. Apply to the hair, starting at about mid-shaft and concentrating down toward the ends. Let the avocado sit on your hair for thirty minutes, and rinse. Voilà! Your hair will feel softer and look shinier, and the avocado will help seal and hydrate those nasty split ends!

FRIZZIES—A BEAUTY NO-NO

For another dry-hair solution, my friend Marlin from Venezuela loves to create her own hair sauna to combat the frizzies that go hand-in-hand with dry hair. One of her favorite secrets is adding a few drops of olive oil to the hair, steering clear of the roots and scalp. After applying, wrap a wet, hot towel around your head for five minutes. Follow with a good shampoo, and you're off to a frizz-free day!

BAT THOSE FABULOUS LASHES

I recently worked with a model by the name of Elisabeth who had the most *amazing* eyelashes. Elisabeth, from Tijuana, told me about a little secret that's not so secret in Mexico. For thick, long, lush lashes, these Mexican beauties use a natural castor oil product called *aceite de ricino,* available in any drugstore in Mexico. These gals end their nightly beauty routine with a swipe of a clean mascara wand dipped in *aceite de ricino.* This is their secret to batting long, lush lashes.

BRAZILIAN CELLULITE FIGHTER

It's common to see Brazilian women, arguably some of the most beautiful women in the world, reclining on the beach rubbing handfuls of sand on their bodies. . . . Why? The coarse sand helps reduce cellulite by smoothing and stimulating the skin, while sloughing off dead cells to reveal fresh skin. How can you go wrong with that?

SMOOTH, FLAWLESS HANDS

The women of Baja give their hands as much attention as the rest of their bodies. For the smoothest, most flawless hands, join these beauties by giving yourself a lemon sugar hand scrub. Mix together 3 tablespoons of white sugar with a few drops of fresh lemon juice. The sugar helps remove dead, dry skin buildup, and the lemon helps fade any unwanted spotting. Beware—this scrub may sting if you have any minor cuts or torn cuticles!

REFRESHING TONER À LA HERBS

In Zacatecas, Mexico, up in the highlands, beauty and nature become one. Because of the arid weather conditions, these beauties must know how to refresh and hydrate their skin. Mint, rosemary, and ginger are some of these gals' favorite herbs. My girlfriend Marcy's family comes from Zacatecas, and she told me that for a refreshing toner, her mom simmers her favorite herbs in water and uses that tea to cleanse and refresh her skin. Try it at home by simmering some of your own favorites like lavender, rosemary, and mint. Let cool. Strain out the herbs and pour the solution into a mister. Spritz it on after you wash your face or throughout the day for a quick pick-me-up! Your refreshed skin will thank you for it.

Beeswax Unwanted Hair

Continuing our journey through Zacatecas, women here love to be fuzz-free. Stubbly legs are a big beauty no-no! Their trick? Beeswax. That's right, they actually melt beeswax and apply it directly on their legs. Then they just peel it off, and remove the excess with a warm cloth. It leaves your legs as smooth and soft as can be!

Antiperspirant the Natural Way

Up in the mountains of Central Mexico, women turn to nature for their antiperspirants. With lemon to combat odor and baking soda to tame perspiration, give this at-home remedy a try.

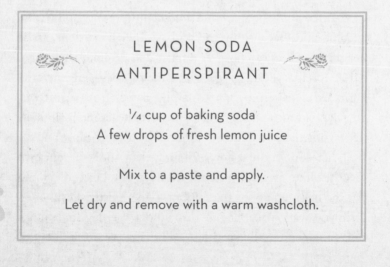

LEMON SODA
ANTIPERSPIRANT

¼ cup of baking soda
A few drops of fresh lemon juice

Mix to a paste and apply.

Let dry and remove with a warm washcloth.

Go Nuts in the Amazon

The women of the Amazon have long been known for their soft, beautiful skin. For centuries these beauties, along with their sister Brazilian tribes, have found softness within the brazil nut. Found in the rain forests of South America, the oil from this "nut" (actually the fruit of a tree) is high in antioxidants and alpha-linolenic acids, which protect and nourish the skin. The Amazonians use this oil as a powerful hair conditioner that strengthens, softens, and adds shine. It also helps to seal the cuticle and helps get rid of split ends. Not to be outdone by other treatments, this miracle oil is also a natural way to moisturize the skin. Acting as a powerful antioxidant, the oil protects the skin from free radicals, hydrates, and helps prevent dryness and flaking, giving the skin an unparalleled, flawless texture. A definite must-have!

Tighten This!

In Baja, California, women have their own secret for a quick facelift. My friend Elizabeth told me about a recipe for a mask passed down by her grandmother. Mix ¼ cup of virgin olive oil (to hydrate and protect the skin) and 1 egg white (to nourish and tighten the skin). Apply this mixture to your face and neck as a mask to help smooth, tighten, and hydrate the skin.

DIET TIPS FROM THE AMERICAS

From the north to the south one thing remains constant: These women are all body conscious and make taking care of their bodies their number one priority. No matter where I went in the Americas, I found that walking was the secret to staying in shape and keeping slim. The beauties told me staying in shape comes down to keeping a good fitness routine and starting their day off at the gym, or at the very least with a morning walk, to keep them looking svelte.

A Midday Feast of Your Favorite Dish

Eat three meals a day and make lunch your heaviest meal. Mexican women start their day with a cup of tea or coffee and a small roll or pastry. Then they eat their biggest meal during lunch. For dinner, they're back to a small a portion to keep up their metabolism.

Orange You Glad for Oranges?

The women in Careyes, Mexico, told me the secret to having a hot body was all in the rind of the orange. Grate the rind of 3 to 4 oranges, mix it with 33 ounces of water, and boil. Then drink a room-temperature glass in the morning, one in the afternoon, and another right before bed. A quick note from these gals . . . it may taste as though you need to add some sugar, but that's a big no-no!

Oatmeal—More Than a Breakfast Treat

One Latin secret to keeping your body regular and lowering your cholesterol is drinking a glass of water with a tablespoon of oatmeal every night before bed. Oatmeal contains a type of fiber that reduces your low-density lipoprotein (LDL), the "bad" cholesterol that can contribute to a higher risk of heart attack and stroke. There's nothing beautiful about being un-healthy!

Linaza for Hair, Linaza for Weight Loss

On my trip through Mexico, I met a beautiful Mexican girl named Daniella Garcia who had the most amazing body! Her secret? Mexican women use a seed called *linaza* for weight loss, as well as keeping beautiful hair. *Linaza* (or flaxseed) is mixed with cold water and taken with breakfast and dinner every day to keep their metabolism up.

Shalini's Beauty Tip

Try using flaxseed oil in your morning smoothies. Blend together your favorite fruits, and add a tablespoon of flaxseed oil. It will keep you satiated, and your skin will look amazing!

SHALINI'S NORTH AND SOUTH AMERICAN MAKEUP TIPS

THE LIPS HAVE IT

If you want to brighten up your look, play up your lips for a change. When visiting Mexico, whether it was north or south, the one thing I noticed about the women was that they all wore lipstick. Even if they had no other makeup on, they would apply a little something on their lips to brighten up their faces. It's a simple trick, with such amazing results. A little color on your lips brightens your entire face! Try the Moroccan Mystique Lip Veils by Global Goddess. They're sheer enough to keep you looking natural but vibrant enough to perk you up instantly!

If you decide to play up your lips, be sure to skip the heavy made-up eyes, and go soft on your cheeks. Make sure to choose a lip color that is soft and not too bright, so that you don't look unfinished. To look like a pro, make sure your brows are groomed, and add a light coat of mascara to frame your eyes. This is one of the quickest ways to look fabulous, fast!

A HEALTHY GLOW

One feature I love about the women in the tropics is their radiant skin. If you don't live in the tropics but want that island glamour, try these tips I use on my clients that you can easily incorporate into your daily beauty routine:

1. Dewy, glowing skin begins with clean skin. Start with a good scrub on your face to slough away dead, dry skin.

2. Follow the exfoliation with a good moisturizer to hydrate and prep the skin for makeup. If you've got oily skin, use an oil-free moisturizer or a mattifying lotion on your T-zone.

3. Invest in a good light-reflecting lotion. This is something that you can find at any drugstore or department store, or you can try the Global Goddess Upgrade Complexion Face Primer with Licorice. It brings a slight shimmer to your face that reflects light. Mix one drop of lotion with your foundation, and apply. Note: If you're trying to get a more youthful look from your makeup, toss your heavy foundation and opt for a lighter, more hydrating texture. Remember, less is more.

4. Apply a gold or pink shimmery crème to your cheekbones, browbone, and down the bridge of your nose. Keep the application light, since the shimmer can be overpowering if you have a heavy hand.

5. Set your look with a triple-milled loose powder. Too much and too heavy a powder will age you and take away the appearance of dewy skin. The silkier the better when it comes to powder shopping. Apply lightly just to set your makeup.

6. Finish with a bronzer by applying it in areas that the sun would naturally hit—your cheeks, temples, chin, and nose. For a more natural look, use bronzer in place of your shadow. The same goes for blush. Instead of your regular blush color, try using bronzer. It will give your skin the instant warmth you've been craving. Try the Global Goddess Goddess Glow South Pacific Shimmer Bronzer.

BRIGHTER AND LIGHTER LOCKS

My girlfriends from South America love to find ways to lighten and brighten their skin tone. One tip they gave me actually had nothing to do with their skin, but more to do with hair. They all swore that lightening their hair created a brightness around their faces that in turn helped them achieve the appearance of lighter skin. It even seemed to take years off their age! I totally agree. As you get older, lighter hair color is more forgiving to the skin than going darker. Also, if you tend to have spotting on the skin or suffer from hyperpigmentation, adding a few lighter strands throughout your hair, especially around the face, will brighten and soften the appearance of any skin issues you might be battling.

6

The Lands
Down Under

n Australia the landscape may be rugged, but women's skin and hair are healthy and smooth. Keeping it natural, they look to the horizon and surrounding lands for hidden gems and coveted beauty secrets. You can bet these Aussie sheilas know that true beauty is as simple as you make it.

Australia may be the smallest continent, but it holds the title of being one of the largest countries on Earth, lying between the Pacific and Indian Oceans in the Southern Hemisphere. The country's capital is Canberra, located in the southeast between the larger and more important economic and cultural centers of Sydney and Melbourne.

Traveling farther through this stunning part of the world, we'll journey to New Zealand to find the reasons that these women have such a healthy glow. Then it's off to paradise in the South Pacific to gather ancient beauty secrets from

DESTINATIONS

Australia, Fiji, New Zealand, Tahiti, and a
quick stop in the South Pacific

some of the most exotic islands in the world. We land in Fiji, where women know that the secrets of anti-aging begin from within. Surrounded by such an exotic landscape, it's their love of life that makes these women emanate internal and external beauty. It's a unique culture of peace and serenity.

LOCAL BEAUTIES

The women down under glow from deep within. This is a destination where nature calls for beauty in simplistic terms. Less is more, and beauty takes its cue from the laid-back lifestyles of the women of Australia, Fiji, and New Zealand. Within these countries women find beauty influences from abroad and learn how to enhance their features without masking their natural beauty. Makeup takes a backseat to a natural, healthy tan, sun-bleached hair, and a bright smile. (They are known to be some of the friendliest people on the planet!)

A TASTE OF THE REGION

Meat pies, bush food (known as bush tucker, these are plants used in jams and chutneys), vegemite (a dark brown vegetable extract spread for bread), and beer make up the traditional meals in Australia. It's a multicultural country, which in turn brings an international flair to the menu by infusing traditional meals with flavors from the East. Australia's own cuisine may be relatively young, but it's evolving quickly. Flavors such as lemon myrtle and Tasmanian peppers are giving Australian dishes their own unique flavor.

Hungry New Zealanders dine on venison and lamb, and are known to have some of the most delicious cheeses in the world. Dinner is considered their heaviest meal, a balanced combination of meat, fish, potatoes, and vegetables.

Fijian Islanders catch fish and dig up root vegetables for staple foods in their diet. One of the unique dishes of Fiji is the *lovo* feast, similar to the Hawaiian luau, that consists of a variety of meats, fish, and vegetables that are packed together, covered with leaves, and cooked in an open pit. Tropical fruits and coconut-based curries with an Indian flair round out the island diet for these gals. And in Fiji, food is traditionally eaten with your fingers. So dig in!

WEATHER REPORT

Seasons in Australia are the opposite of those in America and Europe. The summertime in Australia falls between November and March, while winter is between May and August. Summers in the west can be hot, and as you move north, the weather takes on a tropical feel.

Fiji is sunny year-round—a destination paradise. Australians and New Zealanders flock to these islands around December to avoid the rains and bask in some tropical sun.

BEAUTY SECRETS OF AUSTRALIA AND BEYOND

Rock 'n' Roll, Baby!

As a test of courage and a strong mind, Fijian tribal members used to walk over hot stones. No need to burn your tootsies to reach that state these days. Spas everywhere are cluing in to a special massage technique using warmed stones. Here's how to make your own at-home hot rock massage—a gentler approach to this ancient ritual. Find a few beach stones (ones with smooth, rounded edges), and heat them in a pot of boiling water. Remove the stones carefully and pat dry. Lie down and, with the help of a willing friend, place the stones on your body to release any tension. If you're on your back, try placing them on your stomach, thighs, and shoulders. On your tummy? Then the backs of your knees, your back, and your neck are great spots. For a special treat, take one larger stone and use it to massage coconut oil onto the skin for a full massage. Warning: Be careful the stones aren't too hot. The goal is to relax, not fry. They should be warm, not scalding.

Pure Body Bliss!

It's ultrasmooth, sweet skin the Fijian way! These island women take the sweet, pure cane sugar organically grown in Fiji and mix it with pure coconut oil (rich in vitamins and nutrients, it's a natural replacement for your skin and hair oils) to exfoliate the skin, revealing a more youthful look and feel. It's a sugar high for any skin that needs a quick fix.

TAHITIAN BEAUTIES KNOW BEST

On the shores of Tahiti we find a seductively scented oil called *monoi*—a creation of coconut milk and frangipani flowers soaked together. This rich oil is an ancient Polynesian secret, traditionally used by women to protect their skin and condition their hair. Drench your body and hair in *monoi* to renew and soften your skin. The heady scent will bring a sense of relaxation to a weary mind!

DETOX WITH ALGAE

While in South Asia, I was amazed at how many Fijian-Indians I met there. These are Indian immigrants who for decades have made Fiji their home. Their skin tone is dark and rich—beautiful, to say the least! Of course I took that opportunity to rummage through their beauty bags in search of some island secrets. They mentioned that no spa day is complete without an algae body wrap. Algae from the Fiji Islands contains natural minerals of the sea that break down and detoxify fatty deposits and, at the same time, increase body circulation. Spas in this area of the world use it in body wraps for totally relaxed and pampered skin.

New Skin À la New Zealand

New Zealanders and Aussies know best when it comes to playing with clay. Both of these cultures have been relying on clay's healing properties for centuries—there's even evidence that aborigines used to eat volcanic ash clay to cure a sick stomach! Today's beauty-savvy women in New Zealand look to bentonite clay for numerous skin benefits. Mined in Gisborne on the North Island, at first glance it may seem an unlikely choice for beauty purposes. But this rich gift from the earth is used in spas for back treatments, body wraps, face masks, and hand/foot contour wraps, because of its detoxifying nature. The mud has sulphurous properties (mild exfoliating and calming action) and is used for cleansing and invigorating the skin; it works best on oily skin to tighten pores and help with blemishes. It's also dried and sold as a soap and a mud pack face mask.

Shalini's Beauty Tip

Clay masks are a great way to purify the skin, tighten pores, and absorb oil and dirt. For best results, apply the mask right before you jump into the shower. Allow the steam in the shower to act as a mini facial by opening your pores and giving you maximum purifying benefits.

NEW ZEALAND CURE-ALL

New Zealand *manuka* (similar to the tingly Australian tea tree) can do double duty as a soothing oil or a honey. When the oil is employed, it's first aid for the skin, working as an antifungal during manicures and pedicures or relieving stress and pain during a massage. Turn to the honey, and you'll have found a cure for blemishes, a moisturizing agent for your face, and a natural antioxidant to fight the battle against aging skin. Both *manuka* and tea tree oil are pH-balanced and promote the repair of tissues.

Shalini's Beauty Tip

Don't forget: Such unique ingredients as *manuka* honey can be found at your neighborhood international market or natural health food store. One quick trip and you're ready for global beauty!

THE MIRACLE OF BIG BIRD

Ancient beauty secrets that are tried and true begin with ancient civilizations and, in this case, their fine feathered friends. Beginning in the central desert of Australia some fifty thousand years ago, the aborigines relied on oil from the large emu bird to treat their wounds and burns and to remedy skin ailments. Today's Australians rely on this same oil for deep, penetrating moisture, vitamins, emollients, and amino acids that hydrate even the driest of skin. These stunners also love to use it on their lips and eyes. Emu oil is perfect for those who generally shy away from oil, as it is quickly absorbed, leaves no residue, and works great under your makeup. It also works on skin that is parched, cracked, and has lost its smooth, healthy look. An added benefit? It has been reported that emu oil also thickens aged, mature skin, making it appear younger. One study reported that pure emu oil rubbed onto the skin twice daily would thicken the skin by 14 percent!

ABORIGINAL HEAD MASSAGE

Down in the rugged outback, the natives know a good thing when they see it. The quandong berry, known as the native peach, was traditionally used to nourish hair and heal scalp conditions. Today, it's still used for a penetrating scalp massage, and the fruity aroma is like no other. It will lift your spirits and restore your shine!

Shalini's Beauty Tip

A weekly head massage not only helps stimulate hair growth, but it also helps, relax your body and mind. Make a spa night with a friend. Use your favorite hair oil and massage your worries away while getting thick, shiny hair!

BEE BEAUTIFUL

The buzz down under is bee pollen. On a recent trip, I met a group of Australian women with the most beautiful skin. As it turns out, taking tablets of bee pollen can give you brighter skin and a healthy body. Bee pollen is recognized as one of the most complete foods known to man, with high concentrations of forty-eight vital minerals and vitamins, including iron, protein, calcium, and vitamins A and B. Not only that, but it also has high levels of antioxidants that prevent free-radical damage in joints and cells. Just take a quick buzz over to your local health food store to stock up! Note: Don't use bee pollen if you're allergic to bees or to any type of pollen.

Shalini's Beauty Tip

Always consult your physician before adding any type of supplement or herb to your diet.

SOUR CITRUS FOR SWEET RESULTS

Lemon myrtle, a plant native to Queensland, Australia, has a refreshing scent to its rich pure essential oil. This exquisite essential oil (known to be almost more "lemony" than lemon itself) is used for aromatherapy, vaporization, toiletries, cosmetics, perfumes, and body care products. Research has confirmed this citrus-rich pure essential oil is highly antimicrobial, antibacterial, and antifungal—putting it on the side of great skin and hair.

CLAY YOUR WAY TO CLEAN SKIN

The secret of the New Zealand beauties lies in the white clay. The unique New Zealand halloysite clay (kaolin) is a pure white clay mined at Matauri Bay in Northland. It acts as a molecular sieve on the skin, picking up leftover makeup, pollutants, and dead skin cells.

Shalini's Beauty Tip

When using clay masks to help oily skin and to detoxify, use it no more than 2 to 3 times a week. Overuse can cause dryness and flaking on the skin. It can also cause redness for sensitive skin types.

LATHER UP WITH SPF

Because of Australia's location, it has one of the highest rates of skin cancer in the world. Fortunately, Aussie gals are SPF devotees, realizing the damaging and aging effects of the hot sun. These savvy sun goddesses know to limit their sun exposure during the most damaging times of the day—10 A.M. to 4 P.M. They also know to shield themselves with a sunscreen of at least SPF 15, making sure to reapply throughout the day.

Shalini's Beauty Tip

Traveling to an exotic location? Remember to reapply your sunscreen throughout the day, even if it claims to be sweatproof. Perspiration and humidity can cause the sunscreen to wear off, leaving you vulnerable to sun damage and a nasty sunburn!

CALENDULA—A NEW ZEALAND SECRET

The chemists on my skin-care line couldn't stop raving about the beauty benefits of calendula. Well, looks like the beauties of New Zealand are way ahead of us. They've been using this extract, derived from the dried flowers of golden marigolds, for years. Calendula extract works wonders to soothe inflammation on the skin and mucous membranes. It's an all-out skin saver, reducing body scars, soothing chapped skin, and eliminating broken capillaries. Although it's tough with its healing powers, it's also gentle enough for sensitive skin and for skin that needs a little soothing comfort.

FLAX—MORE THAN A DIET AID

Once used as a healing plant by the Maori, the natives of New Zealand, New Zealand flax now cures all sorts of ailments that today's Kiwi beauties suffer from. A snip of a leaf produces a cooling gel that works its soothing magic on cuts, burns, and sunburns, and for toning the skin. The seed oil is also rich in linoleic acid—perfect for nourishment.

COLD SORES BEGONE!

There's nothing worse than having a hot date or an important meeting and waking up that morning with a cold sore! The women of New Zealand ask Mother Nature for a little help in fighting those pesky sores. New Zealand kanuka oil is very similar to *manuka* but is more antibacterial, attacking cold sores with amazing strength. It's also a much lighter oil than *manuka,* so it won't add a greasy shine.

FUZZY FRUITS WITH HEALING POWERS

The kiwi fruit is one of the most powerful allies you can have against aging skin. It's used throughout New Zealand for all types of skin care. These tiny, fuzzy fruits contain more vitamin C than any other fruit, along with huge quantities of vitamin E, essential fatty acids (such as alpha-linolenic acid), and arginine, which helps stimulate mature skin. The pulp is an amazing antioxidant and antibacterial agent and also has excellent emollient properties.

KIWI MOISTURIZING CLEANSER

1 kiwi fruit
2 tablespoons of plain yogurt
1 tablespoon of orange juice
1 tablespoon of almond oil
1 tablespoon of honey
1 teaspoon of finely ground almonds

Puree the kiwi fruit in a food processor until liquid. While it's processing, add yogurt, juice, almond oil, and ground almonds. Process until thick.

Massage mixture gently over neck, face, and décolletage to cleanse. Rinse well.

Stop Being So Flaky

Eucalyptus makes up nearly 75 percent of Australia's total number of plant species. With its analgesic properties, the oil from this stately plant takes the sting and ouch out of a nasty sunburn. But even better are its benefits to help control those pesky dandruff flakes. Just add a few drops to your shampoo, and wash those flakes away!

Tea Tree Magic

Australian women know that tea tree oil is the solution to all sorts of beauty problems. The oil can bring a youthful glow to tired skin, helping to oxygenate cells and repair damage caused by sun, acne, dry skin, fungus, and other skin disorders. Even those with sensitive skin have given soap with tea tree oil the thumbs-up for effective yet mild cleansing. This tingly oil also works wonders when applied directly to both dandruff and pimples—two tough problems that no beauty wants!

Shalini's Beauty Tip

Tea tree oil works best when mixed with another product. For fighting dandruff, add a few drops to your shampoo. Oily skin? Add a few drops of tea tree oil to your cleanser for an acne-fighting face wash.

Jelly to Firm in No Time

Australian jellybush honey, or *guku,* is a treatment designed to accelerate healing and restore elasticity and firmness to the body. Following a visit to the steam room and a light exfoliation with a loofah, Aussie ladies typically slather on this delicate honey for toning and softening the skin.

Australian Exfoliant for Sensitive Skins

The wattleseed, a funny name but a serious exfoliant kind to your sensitive skin, comes from an indigenous Australian plant. Its unique, round seeds won't scratch the skin's surface. Ground wattleseeds are high in protein and oil, making them an ideal exfoliant for removing dead skin and stimulating cell growth.

Shalini's Beauty Tip

If you have sensitive skin, always look for scrubs that have a gentler granule texture or granules shaped like beads that roll off the skin easily.

Tasmanian Face Lift

The Tasmanian kelp seaweed extract is uniquely Tasmanian and contains minerals and amino acids that stimulate circulation and bring freshness and rejuvenation to the skin. Any face mask or treatment with this unique ingredient is great for dehydrated and mature skin, bringing about a youthful glow and an instant lift.

DIET TIPS OF THE AUSTRALIANS AND BEYOND

A Dehydration No-No

According to my Australian friend Mary O'Malley, water is essential in such a hot, dry country. Drinking water throughout the day not only keeps your body working at its best, but it also keeps your fat burning! Not to mention filling you up for only one serving of shrimp from the barbie!

Take a Hike

The women of New Zealand walk it off. With beautiful scenery and temperate days, these gals use walking, hiking, and bike riding as ways to not only enjoy nature but also to keep their weight in check.

Dance the Night Away

The gals down under are always up for a fun night at the disco. The ones I met said they love to dance the night (and the calories) away. Try incorporating a little dance into your days or nights for a fun, cardio-blasting way to shed pounds. Turn up the hits and bop around as you clean house, prepare a homemade mask in the kitchen, or pick out the perfect outfit for a night on the town.

Love Your Body

This is one of my favorite diet tips because it's not a diet tip at all. It's a lesson in acceptance. Accepting yourself. The Fijian culture teaches women to love their bodies for what they are. Fijian women in particular consider a little weight on a body to be more beautiful. (It's actually taken as a compliment to be told that you're gaining weight.) Until recently, with the introduction of cable TV, Fijian women didn't even consider dieting, which is a nice, welcome change in perspective from our diet-obsessed culture.

MAKEUP TIPS FROM AUSTRALIA AND BEYOND

Women in Australia, New Zealand, and the South Pacific have one thing in common—they keep it natural. They know how to enhance what they were given; they don't mask their features. One thing I love about every woman I meet from down under is their natural glow.

Give Your Best Feature the Spotlight

When making yourself up, do just that—make it yourself. Keep it natural, looking like the real beautiful you. One way to do this is to pick your best feature, and make it stand out. Whether it's your eyes, your lips, or your cheekbones, play it up. Then complement your other features by using shades of neutrals to balance the face. Too much of everything may brighten you up, but will also make you look overdone.

SIMPLIFY YOUR BEAUTY

The stunners down under and in the South Pacific know that ageless beauty is in the hands of sunscreen. Get double duty out of your products and simplify your beauty routine by using moisturizers that contain a minimum of SPF 15. Double up on your makeup by opting for tinted moisturizers that not only cover but also hydrate and protect the skin with a built-in SPF. If you forget to put something on, your other products have got you covered.

MELT-FREE BEAUTY

Because of the hot, humid weather in the South Pacific, it's important for these beauty-conscious women to use makeup that won't melt. Instead of wearing foundation over their entire face, they apply light concealers only in the areas where they need coverage. They then follow with a dusting of loose powder. Waterproof mascara is a definite must, and they finish off their look with a hint of pink gel for a healthy blush.

7

Travel Beauty Essentials

Any seasoned traveler and beauty junkie knows that when you are on the go, the frenzied pace of traveling can make you look less than perfect. Whether you're jetting off to the south of France or just commuting across town to your office, there are rules of play and tricks of the trade that will rescue you from the travel beauty blues!

THE RULES OF FLIGHT

How many times have you walked off a plane to see that your skin looks ten times worse than when you boarded the aircraft? This isn't uncommon, as air travel can take its toll on your hair, skin, and nails. Here are a few tips to keep your skin glowing and to save face—and makeup!

Shalini's Beauty Tip

Pump up your moisturizing routine before, during, and after flying.

GIVE YOUR SKIN A DRINK OF WATER

Dehydration is one of the biggest downsides of travel, especially by air. Recycled air wreaks havoc on your complexion, which is why savvy flight attendants always keep moisturizer on hand and bottled water by their side.

To plump up your skin with moisture before a flight, use a hydrating mask. One secret I share with many of the actors and models I work with is to use a small amount of hydrating mask and sleep with it on the night before you fly. Not only will this give your skin a surge of moisture, but it will also plump up any fine lines. You will awake to a more youthful glow that will last through your time in the air.

Shalini's Beauty Tip

If you have an oily complexion, your skin can still be dehydrated. Exfoliate and then hydrate with an oil-free moisturizer. Remember, you want to add hydration to the skin, which doesn't necessarily mean oil. Try the Global Goddess Ticket to Beauty Flawless Skin series of products. They're everything you need for balanced skin no matter your skin type.

EXFOLIATE FOR BETTER HYDRATION

The most important step in achieving beautiful skin and makeup is to start with well-hydrated skin. To get the most out of your moisturizer, it's important to start your beauty routine with a gentle scrub to exfoliate dead skin. Sloughing off dead skin cells will allow your skin to better absorb your moisturizer as well as allow your makeup to blend seamlessly into your skin instead of sitting on top. I like to keep a gentle scrub in the shower and start my morning with a little scrub-a-dub-dub for an instant glow.

Dewy Skin Equals Beautiful Makeup

One thing I love to do before flying is to mix moisturizer with my foundation for beautiful-looking makeup through-out my trip. Start by mixing one part hydrating serum to one part foundation. Blend well onto your skin. Set your makeup with a triple-milled loose powder. The key to keeping that healthy glow is in keeping your makeup dewy and fresh. That means avoiding products such as heavy powders or matte fin-ishes. When looking for a good quality powder, apply it to the back of your hand. If it blends to an invisible finish and feels silky, then it's the one you're looking for. Avoid powders that leave a white or gray cast and feel gritty. They will add years to your face and give you an ashy finish. Remember, when flying, less is more!

Wake Up Tired Eyes

One big beauty no-no is red, bloodshot eyes. Dry air and a lack of sleep on a flight can irritate your eyes, causing them to look red and swollen, which in turn will add years to your face instantly. Here are some of my favorite rules to play by:

• Avoid black eyeliner and dark shadows. Instead, opt for a navy eyeliner. The blue will brighten up the whites of your eyes. You can also try a deep navy mascara for the same results.

• Keep eye drops or artificial tears on board with you to rehydrate and brighten dry eyes.

• Mix a drop of eye cream with a yellow-based concealer, and apply below your eye area to conceal dark circles, create light reflection, and perk up the appearance of tired eyes.

• Wear a bright pink or peach blush to add color to your face. Stick with a cream formula to keep skin looking dewy.

• Go glossy. Glossy lips are another way to keep lips hydrated, as well as brighten up your over all look.

WHILE YOU'RE IN FLIGHT

H_2O, *eau, acqua, pani, agua por favor.* Translation—water, please! If you're a nervous flyer like me, you automatically reach for the nearest cocktail and then some! Not a good idea unless you want that drink to show up on your face. Alcohol and caffeine add to the already dehydrating effects of flying and can cause facial puffiness. To avoid this, you should double your water intake while flying. For every one cocktail or caffeinated beverage you consume, drink two glasses of water to stay hydrated inside and out. I like to think of this as the 2:1 H_2O factor. I also recommend that all my clients keep water in a spray bottle to periodically mist their faces throughout the flight. It not only refreshes your skin, but it also helps to keep your makeup set, reduce puffiness, and hydrate your face.

ARE WE THERE YET?

Now that you've arrived at your fabulous destination, the last thing you want is to spend time on your beauty routine. You've got sightseeing to enjoy, fruity cocktails to drink, and cultures to explore. Simplicity is the name of the game. Look for ways to simplify your routine and get the most out of your beauty products. Look for products that are multi-use and can be used on more than one feature. Opt for skin care that has a built-in sunscreen. Don't be afraid to play up one feature and bring just enough products to enhance your eyes or your lips or your cheeks. Remember, you're on vacation, baby!

Destination Beauty

Here are a few of my favorite travel essentials that every makeup bag should have:

Tinted moisturizer: It's the easiest way to create an even-looking canvas without feeling like you're wearing a lot of makeup. It's a moisturizer, foundation, and SPF all in one.

Triple crayons: Chubby sticks and multi-use products like lip and cheek stains are a no-brainer. Find products that you can use on your eyes, cheeks, and lips. The less you have to carry, the better.

Pill case: This is one of my favorite tricks. Put all your old lipsticks into a four- or six-compartment pillbox available at any drugstore. This is a great way to make your own lip palette with all your favorite colors. And the best part? You won't have to carry all those half-empty tubes of lipstick!

Lip pencils: Take three of your favorite colors and a clear lip gloss. Once again, cutting down on clutter makes travel so much easier. I suggest a light nude, a medium berry, and a dark crimson, or your favorite color choice. Line and fill in your entire lip. Throw some gloss over the top, and you're off! You get three different looks without packing six or seven different products. The bonus? The lip liner will act as a primer and stay put on your lips. You won't have to worry about losing your lip color or having it fade.

Bronzer: A definite must-have for travel. You can give yourself an allover dust for some warmth, or you can use it as your blush or eye shadow. Depending on your skin color, you can go with anything from a dark bronze (for a dramatic look) to a light, pinky bronze (or more of a healthy glow).

All-in-one makeup palette: If you really want to condense your entire makeup routine into one easy step, invest in a good makeup palette. Most major cosmetic lines carry a face palette with multiple products.

Now to cleanse: I'm a huge fan of cleansing cloths. They are so easy to pack. They cleanse, exfoliate, and hydrate all in one step. And if you use a lot of different moisturizers, the larger version of a four-compartment pillbox is a great way to condense your products for the vacation. Add one moisturizer per compartment, and make sure to label each product and put the pillbox in a Ziploc baggy to avoid any possible spills.

Lip treatment: Nothing says you've been sitting on a plane for hours like chapped lips. A big beauty no-no! I like to apply my lip treatment under my lipstick to keep my lips moist and hydrated through my travels. Make sure to pack a good lip treatment like the Global Goddess Drench Hydrating Lip Spa to not only condition chapped lips, but also to nourish them during the day. I also recommend applying it every night before going to bed. If you're battling severely chapped lips, look into using a lip scrub, or use a wet washcloth and gently scrub your lips. Make sure to always follow any type of exfoliation with hydration.

Hand cream: Don't forget your hands! Applying hand cream before, during, and after the flight will keep your hands hydrated and looking younger. Don't forget to massage some cream onto your cuticles. I don't know about you, but my cuticles crack easily after flying.

Deep conditioner: If you're looking for a good hair day your best bet is packing a deep conditioner to repair the havoc air travel may have caused. Wherever you may be jetting off to, you have no idea how the water, climate, and food are going to affect your hair. Err on the safe side, and keep your hair conditioned and smooth!

Remember, pack light and get the most out of your products!

FAST AND FABULOUS

Now that you have the tools for looking great, do you want to spend an hour in front of the mirror? Most likely you won't have much time but will still want to look put together. Whether it's just a couple of minutes or the luxury of ten, here are a few ways to look fabulous no matter your time constraints!

The Two-Minute Face

Tinted moisturizer: To even out the skin tone, hydrate and protect your skin.

Mascara: Opt for black or navy. Mascara will instantly frame and open up your eyes. If you're in a tropical location, make sure to use a waterproof formula.

Lip gloss: A definite must-have for a sexy pout.

The Five-Minute Face

Crème-to-powder foundation: The perfect way to add a little hydrating color in a jiffy, evening out skin tone and giving you a flawless complexion.

Crème blush: I like a multi-use product that you can use on eyes, cheeks, and lips.

Mascara: Go with a black, plum, or navy to frame and open up your eyes.

Crème shadow: Use a crème formula to "wash" the color across the lid. Try a champagne color for an all-around flattering shade sure to complement any outfit's color scheme. Not only do these crèmes have the versatility of color, but they can be used as a multi-use product—as a hilighter down the bridge of your nose, on your cheekbones, on your browbones, and on the center of your lip for a fuller pout.

Lip gloss: Luscious lips with a sexy glow can pull the entire look together.

THE TEN-MINUTE FACE

Foundation: If you feel like you need extra coverage and have a little extra time, apply a foundation to your problem areas. There's no need to apply it full-face unless you're out for a special occasion and want to look beyond flawless. Also, opt for the travel-friendly crème to powders or stick foundations.

Powder: If you wear foundation, then it's imperative that you set your makeup with a dusting of powder for longer wearability. Use a brush or powder puff and apply lightly, brushing off the excess.

Eye shadow: Start with a "wash" of color across the eyelid. Choose colors that are sheer and neutral for a base shade. Start from the lid, and apply it all the way to the brow.

Apply a deeper shade through the crease to enhance your eye shape.

Mascara: Black will instantly frame and open up your eyes.

Blush: Blush is the quickest way to get some instant color! Warm up your skin and give your cheeks a glow with colors that brighten you up. Try a pink or peach to create a youthful glow on the skin.

Lips: Your choice—lipstick or gloss!

Wherever you go, remember that the more uses you can get out of one product the better, and the fewer products you have to pack, the easier your trip will be.

Bon voyage!

Sources

INTERNET

www.thebodyshop.com

www.taveuni.com.au

www.prweb.com/releases/2002/2/prweb11828.php

www.free-beauty-tips.com

www.touregypt.net/magazine

www.care2.com/healthyliving

www.kitchencraftsnmore.net

www.spaindex.com

www.allnaturalbeauty.us

www.wedmd.com

http://rex.nci.nih.gov/NCI_Pub_interface/rate
risk/rates24.html

PRINT

Shortcuts to Sexy Legs and Butt: 377 Ways to Trim, Tone, Camouflage and Beauty by Cheryl Fenton. Gloucester, MA: Rockport Publishers, 2004.

Naturally Healthy Skin—Tips and Techniques for a Lifetime of Radiant Skin by Stephanie Tourles. Storey Publishing, LLC, 1999.

The Herbal Home Spa: Naturally Refreshing, Wraps, Rubs, Lotions, Masks, Oils, and Scrubs by Greta Breedlove. Storey Publishing, LLC, 1998.

Earth, Water, Fire, & Air by Cait Johnson. Skylight Paths Publishing, 2002.

First Magazine

Index

About the Author

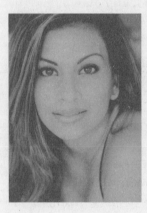

Celebrity makeup artist Shalini Vadhera cannot remember a time when she hasn't been fascinated by the world of beauty. And this fascination has always reached far beyond her own home.

As a first-generation Indian-American, Shalini is no stranger to trips around the globe, with new cultures and histories constantly on her horizon. During her frequent visits to relatives, she would spend hours watching Indian women line their eyes with kohl; wondering at the flawless skin touted by the women of Singapore Airlines and the luxurious hair of Middle Eastern beauties. She began to question—what were the secrets to all of this beauty? It was this international exposure that sparked an enchantment with the beauty techniques of various cultures, and the seed of her lifework was planted.

A self-professed beauty junkie and a celebrity makeup

artist by trade, Shalini knew that she had uncovered something, something that every woman should know—that beauty can be found everywhere. She wanted to bring the fruits of her travels—pearls of beauty wisdom and discoveries of exotic ingredients—to women everywhere.

And Global Goddess Beauty was born—the skin-care and makeup line that helps create awareness of different cultures and countries and all the great beauty secrets they have to offer. With exciting and unique ingredients, combined with fascinating time-tested techniques from generations of women around the globe, Global Goddess Beauty brings the entire world to every woman's doorstep.

Shalini continues to bring this knowledge to her own global television presence as an internationally recognized celebrity makeup artist and global beauty expert for several networks and cosmetics companies.

While completing a degree in international business, Shalini was given the opportunity to work as a makeup artist on NBC's *The Tonight Show* with Jay Leno. After numerous celebrity requests, she went on to work with CBS, Disney, *Hollywood Squares, The Bold and the Beautiful,* the *Survivor* reunions show, and *Dancing with the Stars.* Shalini has also made frequent appearances as a celebrity beauty expert on CBS's *The Early Show,* VH1's *How the Stars Get Hot,* E!'s *Style Star,* Lifetime's *Head to Toe,* TBS's *Movie and a Makeover,* USA's *Before and After'noon Movies, Soap Talk,* Oxygen's *The Isaac Mizrahi Show,* and *Smart Solutions* on HGTV. Her most recent work includes an appearance as a multicultural beauty expert on *Life and Style* and on Entertainment Tonight's *Celebrity Weddings Unveiled* as Hollywood's leading makeup artist.

Shalini also does extensive work as a celebrity makeup artist, boasting a lengthy and impressive client list that includes Alec Baldwin, Brooke Burke, Cybil Shepherd, Simon Cowell, Tyson Beckford, Ty Pennington, and the cast of *The Bold and the Beautiful*.

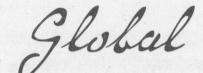

About Global Goddess Beauty

Global Goddess Beauty gives the savvy woman the ticket to ultimate beauty—without leaving her home. It's a beauty adventure around the world, combining the best of tried and true beauty secrets and ingredients from women everywhere.

Global Goddess Beauty unlocks this treasure chest of the best beauty secrets from around the world, bringing you age-old tips and tricks combined with unique and exotic ingredients. Different countries and cultures join in this journey with one goal in mind: a destination of ultimate beauty.

Gathered from her extensive overseas travel, first generation Indian-American Shalini has incorporated beauty secrets from women everywhere into a line of skin care and color that makes leading a glamorous jetset lifestyle an everyday possibility. So, ready, set, jet! It's Destination Glamour.

GLOBAL GODDESS SKINCARE LINE

Global Goddess Skincare guides you along every step of your journey to amazing skin. From washing off the night's slumber to the final intense moisturizing of the day (and all beauty challenges in between), Global Goddess pampers you with unique ingredients from around the world. Beauty adventurers will find their skin glowing from within with Japanese camellia oil; bodies brightened by South Asian turmeric; and faces hydrated with the exotic Spanish prickly pear. Regardless of which global ingredient is your travel companion, flawless skin is your ultimate destination.

GLOBAL GODDESS MAKEUP LINE

Shalini's behind-the-scenes celebrity beauty secrets are revealed within the products of the Global Goddess Makeup Line, along with products that have a multicultural draw. The colors are high in pigment and universally appealing on any complexion, and the line offers core colors that target the tough "mid-range" skin tones, including but not limited to South Asian, Latina, Middle Eastern, and mixed ethnicities. The delicious crème textures are as rich as the finest silk sari, enveloping the skin in first-class luxury, while triple-milled powders disappear quickly to an amazing finish. Global Goddess also tackles multicultural beauty challenges—from false lashes to enhancing Asian eyes to brightening creams for under-eye circles that plague those with darker skin tones. It's a journey through the colors, sites, and sounds of exciting, worldly destinations. The pinks of Jaipur, where Shalini fell in love with the city the King painted pink to impress his dinner guests, to the sands of the Serengeti where Shalini went on her first safari at a young age, Global Goddess Makeup offers a rich palette of color that showcases the beauty that is all around us.

GLOBAL GODDESS PRODUCTS

Passport to Beauty *Skin Essentials*

Shine Coconut Amla Revitalizing Hair Treatment

Ingredients: Coconut oil, henna, and amla extract

Origin: Beauty secret of India

One of the richest oils in the world. Coconut oil is known as a cure-all: It makes hair shiny, strengthens follicles, seals the cuticles, helps with split ends, and stimulates growth. Henna adds volume and shine, and amla extract rejuvenates the scalp.

Seduce White Camellia Face and Body Silk

INGREDIENT: Camellia oil

ORIGIN: Beauty secret of Japan

The high content of oleic acid in this quickly absorbing oil gives it that extra boost to fight most beauty dilemmas—wrinkles, stretch marks, burns, and brittle nails.

Brighten Turmeric Cleansing Body Polish

INGREDIENT: Turmeric, crocus root flower

ORIGIN: Beauty secret of South Asia

Turmeric is a bright orange spice powder with unusual healing properties to soothe, brighten, and create glowing skin. Crocus extract is taken from the white and lavender blooms and assists in the prevention of free-radical damage, which helps to fight aging.

Glow Turmeric Cleansing Face Polish

INGREDIENT: Turmeric

ORIGIN: Beauty secret of South Asia

A bright orange spice powder with unusual healing properties to soothe, brighten, and create glowing skin.

Tighten White Tea Firming Body Quench

INGREDIENT: White tea

ORIGIN: Beauty secret of China

White tea comes from the silver tip of the green tea plant and is one of the strongest antioxidants in the world, helpful in fighting against free radicals.

TICKET TO BEAUTY FLAWLESS SKIN SERIES

Cleanse Dual Face Bath, Erase Brightening Eye Gel

INGREDIENT: Knotweed

ORIGIN: Beauty secret of Japan

Also known as Japanese bamboo or fleece flower, this bamboo-shaped plant houses a high amount of antioxidants to protect and keep the skin radiant.

Refresh Revitalizing Spritzer

INGREDIENT: Prickly pear

ORIGIN: Beauty secret of Spain

The Spanish prickly pear offers intense hydration with its high water content, second only to the cucumber. This rich emollient hydrates and acts as an anti-irritant and moisturizer.

Hydrate Moisture Skin Drink

INGREDIENT: Edelweiss

ORIGIN: Beauty secret of Eastern Europe

Edelweiss is used as an antioxidant to improve the skin's microcirculation and assist in fighting against free radicals; also known to naturally provide UV light–absorbing chemicals.

Drench Hydrating Lip Spa

INGREDIENT: Babassu fruit, buruti fruit, cupuasu fruit

ORIGIN: Beauty secret of the Amazon

Babassu fruit is an oil used as a natural emollient to heal dry skin and leave skin velvety soft. Buruti fruit is rich in vitamin A; oil from this fruit has a rich emollient nature to heal skin and reduce irritation. It's applied to skin and hair for natural protection. Cupuasu fruit, also known as "white cocoa," is extracted from the fruit seeds. This oil is used as a sun protector due to its ability to absorb UV radiation.

COMPLEXION PERFECTION DUO

Foundation/Concealer Duo: Foundation

INGREDIENT: Neem oil, illipe butter, monoi oil

ORIGIN: Beauty secret of India, Africa, and the South Pacific

This rich, fortifying oil extracted from leaves of the neem tree has astringent and purifying properties. It soothes and smoothes skin, especially if you are prone to red, irritated skin, and also can be used to strengthen and repair brittle nails. Illippe nut butter from Africa is highly moisturizing and emollient and helps to nourish and soften the skin. Monoi oil, found in Tahiti, is a creation of coconut milk and frangipani flowers soaked together. This rich oil is an excellent skin softener and is also used to nourish hair.

Foundation/Concealer Duo: Concealer

INGREDIENT: Rose carnina fruit extract, chamomile, lemongrass

ORIGIN: Indonesia, Germany, and Europe

Rose carnina fruit extract is an ultracalming extract that nourishes the skin. Chamomile is a tea used to soothe and soften irritated and dry skin. And lemongrass is an exhilaratingly fragrant herb that acts as an astringent to tighten and lift skin.

GLOBAL GODDESS COLOR LINE AND ACCESSORIES

The Jet Setter Five-Minute Face Case

Upgrade Complexion Face Primer with Licorice (a Russian beauty secret)

BoHo Exotic Eyes Kit

Moroccan Mystique Lip Veils

Goddess Glow South Pacific Shimmer Bronzer

The Jet Setter Mini Tool Case

For more information about these products, please go to www.globalgoddessbeauty.com.